Dictionary of Occupational Therapy

Mark Richard

Table of contents

Activation Level 10
Activity analysis 11
Activity-oriented groups 12
Actuation analysis 14
ADHD 16
Advice on assistive devices 17
Aftercare 19
Animal-assisted therapy 21
Aphasia 23
Apraxia 24
Arthrosis 25
Articulation 27
Athetosis 28
Attention 29
Attention control 30
Autism 31
Back training 33
Balance exercises 35
Basal stimulation 37
Behavioral Analysis 38
Behavioral training 40
Biography work 42
Biomechanics 44

Bobath Concept/Neurodevelopmental Therapy (NDT) 46
Body Awareness 48
Body imago 49
Body Schema 50
Brain Gym 51
Brain Performance Training 52
Case Conference 54
Case Management 56
Case study 58
Caseload 60
Cerebral palsy 61
Chronic illness 63
Chronic polyarthritis/rheumatoid arthritis 64
Cocontraction 65
Cognitive-Behavioral Therapy 66
Communication aids 68
Community Integration 70
Community-Based Rehabilitation 72
Concentration 74
Consultation 75
Contracture 76
Contracture prophylaxis 77
Coordination 79
Coping Strategies 80
Coping with illness 82

Craniosacral Therapy ... 84
Creative Therapy ... 85
Curative Education ... 86
Dementia ... 88
Diabetes management ... 90
Diagnostics ... 92
Differential diagnosis ... 94
Diplegia ... 96
Down syndrome/trisomy 21 ... 97
Dysarthria ... 99
Dyscalculia ... 101
Dyslexia ... 103
Dysphasia ... 105
Dyspraxia ... 107
Early Intervention ... 109
Early rehabilitation ... 111
Endurance training ... 113
Environmental Modification ... 114
Equestrian Therapy/Hippotherapy/Equine-Assisted Therapy (EAT) ... 116
Equilibrium ... 118
Evaluation ... 119
Executive Functions ... 121
Expressive Therapy ... 123
Fine motor skills ... 125

Forearm crutches	127
Frustration tolerance	128
Functional analysis	130
Functional training	131
Gait analysis	133
Geriatrics	134
Gerontology	136
Group therapy	138
Group work	140
Hand Therapy	142
Handcrafts	144
Hand-eye coordination	146
Hemiparesis	148
Hemiplegia	149
Holistic Approach/Holistic Approach	150
Hydrotherapy	152
Hypertension	154
Hypotension	155
Inclusion	156
Increased effectiveness	158
Individual Therapy	159
Instrumental Activities of Daily Living (IADL)	161
Interdisciplinary collaboration	163
International Classification of Functioning, Disability and Health (ICF)	165

Introspection	167
KAWA Model	169
Kinaesthetics	170
Laterality	172
Lifestyle	174
Long-term memory	176
Low Vision	178
Lymphatic drainage	180
Manual Therapy	182
Material Adaptation	184
Medication Management	186
Mentalization	188
Mirror Therapy	190
Motor	191
Motorized planning	192
Multimodal Therapy	194
Music therapy	196
Neurology	198
Neuropsychological Rehabilitation	200
Neuropsychology	202
Nystagmus	204
Orthopaedic technology	205
Orthopaedics	207
OTIPM Model	209
Pain Management	211

Painting Therapy	213
Palliative care	215
Parent Counseling	217
Partial performance fault	219
Patient Counseling	221
Pediatrics	223
PEO Model	225
Perception	226
Perception enhancement	227
Phonological awareness	229
Physiotherapy	230
Pressure ulcer prophylaxis	232
Preventative care	234
Proprioceptive Neuromuscular Facilitation (PNF)	235
Psychiatry	237
Psychoeducation	239
Psychomotor skills	241
Quality management	243
Quality of life	245
Reconstructive Therapy	247
Regulatory disorder	248
Rehab Management	250
Rehabilitation	252
Remotivational Therapy	254
Resilience	256

- Resource orientation ... 258
- Rheumatism ... 260
- Rheumatoid arthritis ... 262
- Self-control ... 264
- Self-management ... 265
- Sensorimotor ... 267
- Sensorimotor integration ... 268
- Sensorimotor skills ... 270
- Sensory Integration Therapy ... 272
- Short ... 274
- Sigmatism ... 275
- Social integration ... 276
- Social reintegration ... 278
- Social Skills ... 280
- Speech therapy ... 282
- Spina bifida ... 284
- Strabismus ... 286
- Stress management ... 287
- Supervision ... 289
- Support Groups ... 291
- Support Reaction ... 293
- Supported communication ... 294
- Tactile ... 296
- Tactile perception ... 298
- Tactile system ... 299

Tetraparesis	301
Tone	302
Tone regulation	303
Transfer Skills	305
Transfer Training	307
Trauma Therapy	309
Treatment plan	311
Tremor	313
Vestibular perception	314
Visual perception	315
Water aerobics	316
Word-finding disorder	317
Youth welfare	318

Activation Level

In occupational therapy, the level of activation refers to a person's level of alertness, attention, and activity. It is an important aspect in the evaluation and planning of occupational therapy interventions, especially in people with various neurological or mental illnesses.

The level of activation can vary from person to person and is influenced by various factors, including physiological, emotional, and environmental factors. An appropriate level of activation is crucial to achieve optimal cognitive and motor function. In occupational therapy, targeted activities and interventions are often used to regulate activation levels.

For example, in people with low levels of activation, occupational therapy can help increase alertness and promote wakefulness through stimulating activities. For individuals with too high a level of activation, relaxation and stress management techniques can be used to support proper regulation.

The individual consideration of the level of activation in occupational therapy work helps to better adapt interventions to the needs of the individual person and to promote the achievement of therapy goals.

Activity analysis

Activity analysis is a central part of occupational therapy practice and refers to the process of detailed examination and evaluation of activities that a person performs in their daily life. The aim is to develop a comprehensive understanding of the person's abilities, limitations and needs in order to then plan and implement targeted interventions.

The activity analysis process can include the following steps:

1. **Identification of the activity:** The first phase involves the selection of the activity to be analyzed. This can be an everyday activity, such as dressing, eating or writing, or even a specific task at work or in your free time.
2. **Decomposition of the activity:** The activity is broken down into its individual components or steps. This allows for a detailed examination and evaluation of the motor, cognitive, sensory, and emotional demands of each component.
3. **Skills assessment:** The analysis involves assessing the individual's abilities in relation to each activity component. This may include skills in fine and gross motor skills, cognitive function, perception, endurance, and other relevant aspects.
4. **Identification of limitations:** It identifies possible limitations or barriers that could prevent the person from successfully performing the activity.
5. **Development of interventions:** Based on the activity analysis, targeted occupational therapy interventions are developed to improve skills, overcome barriers and promote the person's independence and quality of life.

Activity analysis is a dynamic process that adapts to the individual needs of the person. It plays a crucial role in the holistic planning and implementation of occupational therapy measures.

Activity-oriented groups

Activity-oriented groups in occupational therapy refer to group activities or programs that aim to engage participants in meaningful and purposeful activities. These groups are often led by occupational therapists and are designed to develop participants' social, emotional, cognitive, and physical skills. The focus is on the use of activities as a means to achieve individual goals and improve quality of life.

Activity-oriented groups include:

1. **Targeted activities:** The group activities are selected to meet the needs and goals of the participants. This can range from handicraft activities to creative projects and joint leisure activities.
2. **Fostering skills:** Activity-oriented groups provide an opportunity to develop and improve various skills, including motor, cognitive, social, and emotional skills. The selection of activities can be tailored to the specific needs of the group members.
3. **Social interaction:** Participating in group activities encourages social interactions. This is especially important for people who need social support or have difficulties with social participation.
4. **Community and belonging:** Activity-oriented groups often create a supportive community and foster a sense of belonging. This is especially relevant for people who feel isolated or have difficulty socializing.
5. **Quality of life and well-being:** By encouraging meaningful activities, activity-oriented groups help improve participants' quality of life and overall well-being. Activities can provide joy and fulfillment.
6. **Evaluation and adjustment:** Occupational therapists regularly monitor and evaluate group members' participation and progress. This makes it possible to customize the activities and ensure that they meet individual needs.

Activity-oriented groups can take place in a variety of settings, such as care facilities, rehabilitation centres, psychosocial settings or community centres. They provide a supportive environment where people can improve their skills, socialize and improve their quality of life through meaningful activities.

Actuation analysis

Activity analysis is a central concept in occupational therapy and refers to the systematic study and evaluation of the activities or activities that a person performs in their daily life. Occupational therapists use activity analysis to understand a person's individual activity level, abilities, limitations, preferences, and goals. This process makes it possible to develop tailor-made interventions to improve independence and quality of life.

Here are some key elements of actuation analysis:

1. **Identification of activities:** Occupational therapists analyze a person's daily activities, whether it is dressing, eating, locomotion, leisure activities or professional activities. These pursuits may include basic activities of daily living (ADL), productive activities, or leisure activities.
2. **Skills and limitations:** Activity analysis assesses a person's abilities and limitations in relation to certain activities. This can include physical, cognitive, emotional, or sensory aspects.
3. **Environmental factors:** The analysis takes into account the environment in which the activities take place. These include physical environmental factors such as housing or workplace, social support systems, cultural aspects, and other external influences.
4. **Personal goals and preferences:** The activity analysis takes into account the individual goals and preferences of the person. This helps to design a therapy tailored to the needs and desires of the individual.
5. **Analytical and holistic perspective:** Activity analysis is carried out both on an analytical level, by looking at specific components of an activity, and on a holistic level, in order to understand the overall context and interactions.
6. **Observation and interviewing:** Occupational therapists use observational techniques and interviews to gather information for activity analysis. This can include directly observing an activity, interviewing the person, or even talking to relatives or caregivers.

The results of the actuation analysis serve as the basis for the development of an individual treatment plan. This plan may include various interventions aimed at improving or adapting the activities in question in order to promote the person's independence and quality of life.

ADHD

ADHD stands for Attention Deficit Hyperactivity Disorder. It is a neurobiological developmental disorder that manifests itself mainly in childhood, but can also persist in adulthood. The disorder is characterized by problems with attention, impulsivity and hyperactivity.

The three main characteristics of ADHD are:

1. **Attention problems:** Difficulty maintaining attention for long periods of time, being easily distracted, and managing organizational tasks.
2. **Impulsivity:** Impulsive behavior that often leads to actions being carried out without sufficient consideration. This can lead to social difficulties and rash actions.
3. **Hyperactivity:** Excessive physical restlessness and impulsivity, which can manifest itself in restless behavior, excessive talking, and difficulty sitting quietly.

Occupational therapists play a crucial role in treating people with ADHD by helping them develop self-regulation strategies, improve their attention, and develop their motor skills. Therapy can aim to improve people's daily functions and quality of life by taking into account their individual needs and challenges.

Advice on assistive devices

Assistive Device Counseling refers to professional advice and support in the selection and use of assistive devices designed to help people with special needs. This counselling can take place in a variety of contexts, including medical care facilities, rehabilitation facilities, specialist counselling centres or in the home environment. The counselling for assistive devices includes:

1. **Needs assessment:** A central task of assistive device counselling is the precise assessment of the person's needs. This includes identifying the nature and severity of the impairment, as well as analysing the day-to-day activities where assistance is needed.
2. **Selection of suitable aids:** Based on the assessment of needs, assistive technology consultants recommend suitable aids. These may include technological devices, adapted tools, mobility aids, communication aids, orthopaedic aids or other specific devices.
3. **Customization and individualization:** Assistive technology counselors can tailor assistive devices to the individual's individual needs and abilities. This may include the selection of special sizes, settings or adjustments.
4. **Instruction and training:** In addition to assisting with the selection process, the consultants also provide training on the proper use of the aids. This may include the correct use, maintenance and care of the assistive devices.
5. **Information about financing options:** Aids can be costly. The advisors inform users about financing options, insurance benefits and subsidy programs in order to minimize costs.
6. **Advice on barrier-free remodeling:** In some cases, it may be necessary to adapt the home environment to facilitate the use of assistive devices. Assistive technology consultants provide recommendations for barrier-free adaptations.
7. **Ongoing support:** The needs of people with special needs can change over time. Assistive Device Counseling provides ongoing support to ensure that the chosen aids meet changing needs.

8. **Collaborating with other professionals:** Assistive counselors often work with other health care providers, therapists, doctors, and social workers to ensure comprehensive care.

Assistive device counselling is important to ensure that people with special needs have access to the appropriate tools to improve their independence, mobility and quality of life. It is an individualized process that is tailored to each individual's unique needs and goals.

Aftercare

Aftercare refers to the continued care and support of individuals after they have completed medical treatment, therapy, or intervention. This phase of care is crucial to maintain the success of the previous actions, prevent possible relapses and ensure that the person continues to take optimal care of their health and well-being. Aftercare is important in various areas of health care and social support. Some features of aftercare include:

1. **Medical Aftercare:**
    - After medical treatments such as surgeries, procedures or hospitalizations, continuous medical monitoring and care is often necessary to follow the healing process and detect any complications at an early stage.
2. **Therapeutic aftercare:**
    - After completing a therapeutic intervention, such as psychotherapy, physical therapy, or rehabilitation, follow-up may include continuations of therapy sessions or monitoring progress to ensure goals are met.
3. **Medication follow-up:**
    - Individuals taking medications may need regular monitoring, dosage adjustments, and evaluation of efficacy to ensure medication continues to be appropriate.
4. **Addiction Aftercare:**
    - After addiction therapy or weaning, follow-up care is crucial to prevent relapses. It may include support through support groups, therapy, or specialized programs.
5. **Health promotion and prevention:**
    - Follow-up care often includes measures to promote healthy behaviors and prevent relapses or new health problems. This may include lifestyle changes, nutritional counseling, or fitness programs.

6. **Psychosocial support:**
    - Aftercare often includes psychosocial support, whether through professional counseling, group therapy, or social services. This can help deal with the emotional and social impact of health issues.
7. **Family and family support:**
    - In some cases, it is important to involve family members or caregivers in aftercare to create a supportive environment and facilitate the transition to normal living.
8. **Monitoring of side effects:**
    - Follow-up care involves continued monitoring for possible side effects of treatments, especially with long-term or repeated therapies.

Follow-up care should be considered an integral part of any treatment plan to ensure that the progress made is sustainable and supports the person's long-term health and quality of life. The specific follow-up measures vary depending on the type of disease, therapy or intervention.

Animal-assisted therapy

Animal-assisted therapy is a form of therapy in which animals are used as part of the therapeutic process to promote the physical and emotional health of humans. This therapy can be used in a variety of settings, including hospitals, nursing homes, schools, and therapeutic practices. Here are some important aspects of animal-assisted therapy:

1. **Goals of therapy:**
   - Animal-assisted therapy has different goals, depending on the needs of the participants. These include improving physical health, emotional stability, social skills, communication, and cognitive function.
2. **Use of animals:**
   - Animals used in animal-assisted therapy can include dogs, cats, horses, birds, rabbits, and other animals. The choice of the animal depends on the goals of the therapy and the needs of the participants.
3. **Therapeutic activities:**
   - Activities in animal-assisted therapy vary depending on the type of animal and the goals of the therapy. This includes petting, feeding, grooming, walking or riding horses.
4. **Stimulation of emotions:**
   - The presence of animals can elicit a positive emotional response. Animals are often perceived as supportive, comforting, and non-judgmental, which can promote emotional well-being.
5. **Physical Benefits:**
   - Interacting with animals can also have physical benefits, such as improving fine motor skills, promoting flexibility, and strengthening muscles.
6. **Social Interaction:**
   - Animals can serve as intermediaries for social interactions. People who have difficulty building

social relationships may be motivated to interact with others by the presence of an animal.
7. **Therapeutic environments:**
   - Animal-assisted therapy can be performed in a variety of therapeutic settings, including working with psychologists, occupational therapists, physical therapists, or teachers.
8. **Applications in various areas:**
   - Animal-assisted therapy has applications in various fields, including the treatment of mental illness, autism, trauma, physical disabilities, and developmental disorders.
9. **Training of Therapy Animals:**
   - Animals used in animal-assisted therapy undergo special training to ensure that they are well prepared to interact with humans.
10. **Ethics and Standards:**
    - There are ethical guidelines and standards for animal-assisted therapy to ensure that the welfare of animals and participants is protected.

Animal-assisted therapy should be carried out by qualified professionals who are trained in both the field of therapy and the handling of animals.

Aphasia

Aphasia is an acquired language disorder that develops due to damage to the area of the brain responsible for language production and processing. This damage can be caused by strokes, brain injuries, tumors, or other neurological disorders. Aphasia affects a person's ability to understand, speak, read, or write language.

There are different types of aphasia, and symptoms can vary depending on the type and location of the brain damage. The most common types of aphasia include:

1. **Broca's aphasia (non-fluent aphasia):** In this form, speech production is impaired while speech comprehension skills are largely preserved. Sufferers have difficulty speaking fluently and may have problems with grammar and word finding.
2. **Wernicke's aphasia (liquid aphasia):** Here, the ability to understand speech is impaired while speech production remains fluent. However, the utterances may be meaningless or incoherent. Sufferers have difficulty understanding the content of their own language and often output words that do not make sense.
3. **Global aphasia:** This form is more severe and significantly affects both speech production and comprehension. Sufferers have difficulty expressing themselves verbally, understanding words, reading or writing.
4. **Amnestic aphasia:** This is a mild form of aphasia in which word recognition is impaired. Sufferers may have difficulty recalling words, although their speech production may otherwise be normal.

Rehabilitation for aphasia often involves speech therapy, in which targeted exercises are performed to improve language skills. The therapy can be tailored to the individual needs and difficulties of the affected person. Early intervention is often crucial to achieve the best outcomes. Aphasia does not necessarily affect a person's cognitive abilities, many people with aphasia retain their intellectual abilities despite the language difficulties.

Apraxia

Apraxia is a neurological disorder that affects a person's ability to perform purposeful and coordinated movements, despite the fact that the motor and sensory functions themselves are intact. This impairment often affects complex actions and motor processes, such as putting on clothes, eating with cutlery or using tools.

There are several forms of apraxia, including ideomotor apraxia, in which the ability to perform motor actions in response to verbal prompts is impaired, and ideatory apraxia, in which the understanding of the purpose of actions or the ability to plan actions may be impaired.

The causes of apraxia can be varied, including damage to specific areas of the brain, especially the parietal and frontal regions. Treatment of apraxia is often carried out through occupational therapy interventions, which aim to restore or compensate for motor skills and improve the quality of life of those affected.

Arthrosis

Osteoarthritis, also known as degenerative joint disease or joint wear and tear, is a chronic condition characterized by the progressive breakdown of cartilage in the joints. Cartilage is the smooth, elastic tissue that covers the ends of the bones in a joint and acts as a shock absorber and lubricant. When cartilage decreases, the bones rub directly against each other, which can lead to pain, inflammation, and loss of function.

Some notable features of osteoarthritis include:

1. **Pain:** Pain is common, especially when the affected joint is loaded. The pain can develop insidiously and increase over time.
2. **Stiffness:** The mobility of the joint may be limited, especially after prolonged periods of rest. Morning stiffness is also common.
3. **Swelling:** Inflammation can lead to swelling in the affected joint.
4. **Changes in joint shape:** As osteoarthritis progresses, changes in the shape of the joint can occur, such as ankle growths (osteophytes).
5. **Loss of function:** Osteoarthritis can affect the function of the affected joint and make everyday activities difficult.

The exact causes of osteoarthritis are not always clear-cut, but they can include a combination of genetic, mechanical, metabolic, and age-related factors. Joint strain, obesity, genetic predisposition, injuries and certain diseases can increase the risk of developing osteoarthritis.

Treatment of osteoarthritis is aimed at relieving pain, improving joint function and slowing down the course of the disease. Therapeutic approaches include:

1. **Drug therapy:** Painkillers, anti-inflammatory drugs, and in some cases, injections may be prescribed.

2. **Physical therapy:** Exercises to strengthen muscles and improve joint mobility are important.
3. **Weight management:** If you are overweight, reducing your body weight can reduce stress on your joints.
4. **Surgical intervention:** In advanced cases, joint replacement surgery (arthroplasty) may be considered.

The treatment of osteoarthritis should be individually tailored to the needs of the patient. Early diagnosis and a holistic approach can help alleviate symptoms and improve quality of life.

Articulation

Articulation refers to the ability to form sounds and pronounce them clearly. It is an essential part of verbal communication. Effective articulation allows a person to express sounds, words, and phrases in a way that can be understood by others.

Articulation disorders can occur when a person has difficulty forming certain sounds correctly. These disorders can be caused by a variety of causes, including:

1. **Phonological disorders:** problems with the organization of sounds in the speech system.
2. **Motor disorders:** Difficulty with the motor movements required for articulation.
3. **Organic causes:** abnormalities or injuries to the anatomical structures involved in speech.

Articulation disorders can refer to individual sounds or groups of sounds. Some children may have difficulty articulating certain sounds as part of normal language development, while others may have difficulties.

Treatment of articulation disorders is often provided by speech therapy intervention. The therapist works to promote the correct articulation of the sounds by using specific exercises and techniques. Therapy can vary depending on the individual needs of the patient.

Certain variations in articulation may be normal, especially in the early stages of language development. However, if articulation disorders persist longer than expected or significantly affect intelligibility, it is advisable to seek professional help.

Timely diagnosis and intervention can help improve articulation disorders and positively influence language development.

Athetosis

Athetosis is a neurological movement disorder characterized by slow, involuntary, snake-like, and writhing movements of the extremities. These movements are usually slow and fluid, as opposed to fast, jerky movements that can occur with other movement disorders such as choreoathetosis.

The causes of athetosis can be varied and include damage or abnormalities in certain areas of the brain, especially in the basal ganglia system, which plays a central role in motor control. Athetosis often occurs in conjunction with other neurological disorders, such as cerebral movement disorders.

People with athetosis may have difficulty holding objects, writing, or performing other fine motor tasks. Symptoms can change over time and vary in severity.

Treatment for athetosis usually focuses on treating the underlying cause, relieving symptoms, and promoting the sufferer's functional independence. Physical therapy, occupational therapy, and other rehabilitative approaches can be part of the treatment plan to improve movement skills and increase quality of life.

Attention

Attention is the ability to consciously and purposefully focus on specific stimuli or information. It is a complex cognitive process that allows us to select and process from the multitude of sensory impressions those that are relevant to our current task or situation.

There are several points of attention:

1. **Selective attention:** The ability to focus on a specific task, stimulus, or source of information while blanking out irrelevant information.
2. **Divided attention:** The ability to focus attention on multiple stimuli or tasks at the same time. It includes the ability to switch back and forth between different activities.
3. **Sustained attention (perseverance):** The ability to maintain attention for long periods of time, especially during repetitive or lengthy tasks.
4. **Changing attention:** The ability to switch between different tasks or sources of information without sacrificing efficiency or accuracy.
5. **Selective Sustained Attention:** The ability to focus attention on a specific task or stimulus for an extended period of time, despite distracting influences.
6. **Attention control:** The ability to flexibly control and adjust attention according to the demands of the situation at hand.

Problems with attention can occur with various neurological or psychological conditions, including attention deficit hyperactivity disorder (ADHD), depression, stroke, or other neurological conditions.

Attention plays a crucial role in daily life, whether it's studying, working, trafficing, or social interactions. Strategies to promote attention may include cognitive training programs, behavioral interventions, adjustments to the environment, or medication approaches, depending on the underlying cause and individual needs.

Attention control

Attention directing refers to the process of directing or focusing a person's attention on specific stimuli, information, or tasks. This process is crucial for the cognitive processing of information and the successful completion of tasks in everyday life. The ability to direct attention varies from person to person and can be influenced by various factors.

Some important information about attention control:

1. **Selective attention:** The ability to focus on certain stimuli or information while ignoring others. This makes it possible to process information in a targeted manner in an environment with many stimuli.
2. **Divided attention:** The ability to focus attention on multiple stimuli or tasks at the same time. This is important in order to handle different requirements at the same time.
3. **Sustained attention:** The ability to maintain attention for long periods of time, especially during repetitive or prolonged tasks.
4. **Flexibility of attention:** The ability to flexibly shift attention between different tasks or tasks, depending on the demands of the situation.

Effective attention control is important for many areas of life, including academic or professional performance, social interactions, and personal organization. In people with attention deficit disorders, such as ADHD, attention control may be impaired, leading to difficulty concentrating and self-regulating.

Strategies to improve attention control may include cognitive therapy, behavioral interventions, specific exercise programs, and, in some cases, drug treatment. These approaches can help strengthen attention skills and make it easier to cope with daily demands.

Autism

Autism, also known as autism spectrum disorder (ASD), is a neurodevelopmental disorder that can affect social interaction, verbal and nonverbal communication, and repetitive behavior to varying degrees. Autism is referred to as the spectrum because the severity and severity of symptoms can vary significantly from person to person.

Some common features of autism include:

1. **Social challenges:** Difficulty establishing and maintaining social relationships, difficulty interpreting social signals, and limited social interests.
2. **Communication difficulties:** Impairments in verbal and non-verbal communication, such as difficulty making eye contact, limited gesticulation, and difficulty understanding irony or sarcasm.
3. **Repetitive behavior:** Repetitive actions, stereotypical movements, or fixed interests may be more common in people with autism.
4. **Sensory sensitivity:** Sensitivity to certain sensory stimuli, such as light, sound, or touch.
5. **Limited interests:** Intense fixation on certain topics or activities, as well as difficulty sharing interests with others.

Autism is usually diagnosed in the first few years of life, as symptoms become apparent in early childhood. Early intervention and individual support are important to improve the quality of life of people with autism and promote their integration into society.

It should be emphasized that autism encompasses a wide variety of individual abilities, talents, and challenges. The term "spectrum" emphasizes the diversity and uniqueness of each individual with autism.

The exact causes of autism are not fully understood, but a combination of genetic, neurological, and environmental factors is suspected. Early interventions, including behavioral therapy, speech therapy support, and supportive education, can have a positive impact on the development of people with autism. Their individual needs should be identified and appropriate support provided.

Back training

Back training refers to targeted exercises and activities aimed at strengthening the muscles in the back, improving posture and preventing back pain. A well-performed back workout can help improve the flexibility of the spine, stabilize the muscles, and strengthen the entire back area. Here are some characteristics of back training:

1. **Strengthening of the back muscles:**
   - Targeted exercises that focus on the muscles in the upper, middle, and lower back are performed to increase the stability and strength of these muscle groups.
2. **Core muscle training:**
   - An important part of back training is training the core muscles, including abdominals, lateral core muscles, and deeper back muscles. Strong core muscles support the spine and improve posture.
3. **Flexibility exercises:**
   - Stretching exercises are incorporated to improve the flexibility of the muscles and promote the freedom of movement of the spine.
4. **Posture training:**
   - Back training often involves exercises aimed at improving posture. This includes awareness of a neutral spinal position and training to maintain this posture in everyday life.
5. **Attention to the spinal load:**
   - During back training, care is taken to minimize strain on the spine. This includes correct lifting techniques and avoiding movements that can cause excessive pressure on the spine.
6. **Full body workout:**
   - Back training is often part of a holistic approach that also involves other muscle groups. A balanced workout promotes overall body fitness and helps prevent muscle imbalances.

7. **Strengthening of the core muscles:**
   - The muscles of the trunk area, including the lateral abdominal muscles and the back extensors, are strengthened to support the stability and alignment of the spine.
8. **Progressive Training:**
   - Back training can be progressively designed by gradually increasing the intensity, number of repetitions and complexity of the exercises. This promotes a gradual improvement in back strength and endurance.
9. **Coordination and Balance:**
   - Exercises to improve coordination and balance are integrated into the training. This promotes proprioceptive abilities and supports the stability of the spine.
10. **Customization:**
    - Back training should be tailored to individual needs and fitness levels. Personalized training takes into account possible limitations or specific back problems.

People with existing back problems should seek professional advice before starting a back training program. Back training can be done as a standalone program or as part of a broader fitness plan to promote overall back health.

Balance exercises

Balance exercises play an important role in the occupational therapy context, especially when it comes to improving functional mobility and safety in everyday life. Occupational therapists use targeted exercises to help people develop or regain their balance and coordination, whether due to injury, neurological conditions, or other health conditions. Here are some examples of balance exercises in an occupational therapy context:

1. **Standing with your eyes closed:**
   - The patient stands with their eyes closed to minimize visual input and increase dependence on the sense of balance.
2. **Coordination of head and eye movements:**
   - The patient performs head movements in conjunction with eye movements to improve head-eye coordination, which is important for balance.
3. **Balance training on unstable surfaces:**
   - The use of unstable underlays such as balance pads, unstable platforms or air cushions can challenge and improve the feeling of balance.
4. **Exercises on one leg:**
   - Standing on one leg or performing movements, such as lifting the knee or bending the ankle, can promote stability and balance.
5. **Exercises with different viewing directions:**
   - The patient performs balance exercises while turning his head in different directions or raising and lowering his gaze.
6. **Dynamic Balance Exercises:**
   - Occupational therapists often incorporate dynamic movements such as walking on a narrow beam, walking sideways, or moving through obstacles.
7. **Transfer exercises:**
   - Exercises aimed at coping with transfers, such as getting out of a chair or crossing doorsteps, can promote balance in everyday situations.

8. **Sensorimotor integration:**
    - The integration of sensory stimuli, such as tactile or vibrational stimuli, can improve the body's perception and response to the ground.

The choice of exercises is made individually, depending on the needs and goals of the patient. The occupational therapist adapts the exercises to the specific challenges of the individual and works towards integrating the acquired skills into everyday life. The holistic approach of occupational therapy takes into account not only the physical, but also the cognitive and psychosocial aspects of balance.

Basal stimulation

Basal stimulation is a concept used in occupational therapy and nursing, especially in the care of people with severe disabilities or limitations. The concept was developed by the German pedagogue and special education teacher Andreas Fröhlich.

Basal stimulation aims to promote perception, motor skills and communication in people with severe impairments through targeted sensory stimuli. Different senses such as the sense of touch, balance and the proprioceptive sense are addressed. Through targeted touches, movements and other stimuli, basic experiences are to be made possible and perception skills are to be improved.

The application of basal stimulation is done individually, based on the needs and abilities of the individual. This can include, for example, the use of special materials, adapted movement exercises or multi-sensory approaches. The aim is to improve the quality of life of the person concerned, to promote their independence and to enable them to participate meaningfully in everyday life. Basal stimulation is often used in working with people with severe mental or physical impairments, as well as in neurological diseases or in the field of geriatrics.

Behavioral Analysis

Behavioral analysis is a systematic approach to studying and modifying behavior. It is based on the principles of behavioral psychology and is applied in various disciplines, such as psychology, pedagogy, organizational development, and therapy. Key features of behavioral analysis are:

1. **Principles of Conduct:**
   - Behavioral analysis uses basic principles of behavioral psychology, including stimulus-response associations, positive and negative reinforcement, punishment, extinction, and the idea that behavior is influenced by its consequences.
2. **Functional Analysis:**
   - An important part of behavioral analysis is functional analysis. This investigates why certain behaviors occur by looking for the conditions that reinforce or weaken the behavior.
3. **Antecedents and consequences:**
   - Behavioral analysis looks at both the antecedents (triggers) and the consequences of behavior. The antecedents are events or circumstances that precede a behavior, while the consequences are the response to the behavior.
4. **Positive Reinforcement:**
   - Positive reinforcement refers to the application of a positive stimulus or reward to reinforce a desired behavior and increase the likelihood of it occurring again.
5. **Negative Reinforcement:**
   - Negative reinforcement refers to the removal or avoidance of an unpleasant stimulus in order to reinforce a desired behavior.
6. **Punishment:**
   - Punishment refers to the application of a negative stimulus to reduce the likelihood of an undesirable behavior occurring again.

7. **Extinction:**
   - Extinction refers to the process by which a behavior decreases or disappears because it is no longer reinforced.
8. **ABA (Applied Behavior Analysis):**
   - ABA is a special application of behavioral analysis that is applied to practical situations and problems. It is widely used in the therapy of autism spectrum disorders (ASD), but can also be used in other contexts, such as pedagogy and organizational development.
9. **Ethics:**
   - Behavioral analysis follows ethical guidelines to ensure that interventions are respectful, effective, and responsible. Adherence to ethical standards is crucial to protect the well-being of those affected.

Behavioral analysis is a flexible approach that can be tailored to different situations and individuals. It is used both to modify undesirable behavior and to promote positive behaviors.

Behavioral training

Behavioral training refers to a pedagogical approach that aims to modify or improve behavior by using specific techniques and strategies. This approach is used in various contexts, including education, workplace, psychology, and therapy. The main goal of behavioral training is to promote desirable behavior and reduce or eliminate undesirable behavior.

Learn more about behavioral training:

1. **Setting goals:** Clear goals are defined before behavioral training begins. These goals can target both the positive behaviors to be encouraged and the undesirable behaviors to be reduced.
2. **Positive reinforcement:** Behavioral training often makes use of positive reinforcement, in which positive consequences are added to reinforce desired behavior. This can be in the form of praise, rewards, or other positive stimuli.
3. **Negative reinforcement:** This is the removal or reduction of an unpleasant stimulus in order to reinforce desired behavior. Negative reinforcement should not be confused with punishment; it is about ending or avoiding an unpleasant state in order to encourage the desired behavior.
4. **Punishment:** In some cases, punishment can also be used as a technique to reduce undesirable behavior. It is important that punishment is appropriate and fair, and that positive reinforcement is preferred to create positive incentives to learn.
5. **Model learning:** Observing and mimicking role models can be an effective part of behavioral training. By exhibiting desired behavior, others can learn how to behave appropriately in certain situations.
6. **Clear instructions and expectations:** Clear communication of expectations and instructions is crucial. The people who do the behavioral training need to make sure that the behaviors to be changed are clearly understood.

Behavioral training is widely applied in schools, businesses, therapeutic settings, and other contexts where it is important to guide and shape the behavior of individuals in order to achieve positive outcomes. A respectful and positive approach is often more effective than using punishment techniques exclusively.

Biography work

Biography work is a method used in various social and therapeutic contexts, including occupational therapy. It refers to the systematic examination of a person's life history in order to gain insights into their experiences, developments, and resources. Life history analysis can be used to strengthen identity, promote self-understanding, and plan therapeutic interventions.

Here are some key aspects of biography work:

1. **Recording of life history and events:** This includes the systematic collection of information about the course of life, significant events, key experiences, relationships and developments.
2. **Biographical interviews:** Biography work often involves conducting biographical interviews in which the person talks about different stages of life and experiences. This not only promotes remembrance, but also allows for a dialogue about personal history.
3. **Reflection and processing:** The person reflects on the events they have experienced together with a therapist or supportive person. This can help to process emotions, to recognize contexts of meaning and to identify patterns in one's own life story.
4. **Resource orientation:** Biography work focuses on identifying resources, strengths, and successful coping strategies that have been used in the past. These can be used as a basis for the development of action strategies in the present.
5. **Identity strengthening:** By engaging with one's own biography, people can strengthen their identity and develop a better understanding of their personality, values, and goals.
6. **Application in occupational therapy:** In occupational therapy, biography work is used to individualize the therapy process. Knowing the person's life history helps to understand the person's needs, goals, and preferences and to choose appropriate interventional approaches.

Biography work is applied in various settings, including nursing homes, psychiatric care, rehabilitation and palliative care. It can help to strengthen the therapeutic relationship, promote self-understanding and support the personal development process.

Biomechanics

Biomechanics is an interdisciplinary field that applies the principles of mechanics to biological systems. Biomechanics studies the structure, function and movement of living organisms, especially the human body. The goal is to understand the mechanisms underlying the movements and forces in biological systems. In occupational therapy and other health professions, biomechanics plays an important role in assessing movement, developing treatment plans, and preventing injuries.

Here are some features of biomechanics:

1. **Kinetics and kinematics:** Kinetics deals with the forces acting on the body, while kinematics looks at the motion itself, independent of the forces. Both aspects are crucial for understanding the movements in the human body.
2. **Musculoskeletal system:** Biomechanics analyzes the structure and function of the musculoskeletal system, including the bones, muscles, tendons, and joints. This is important for understanding movements, joint stability, and the distribution of forces during movement.
3. **Gait analysis:** Biomechanical principles are used in gait analysis to understand the normal or aberrant movement patterns when walking. This is especially relevant in rehabilitation and orthopedics.
4. **Stress and deformation:** Biomechanics looks at the effects of stress and deformation on biological structures. This is essential for the prevention of injuries and the development of therapeutic approaches.
5. **Ergonomics:** Ergonomics, a field of biomechanics, studies how the interaction between people and their environment can be designed to improve the efficiency and safety of work processes.
6. **Sports biomechanics:** Biomechanics is also used in sports to analyze athletes' movements, optimize performance, and prevent injuries.

In occupational therapy, the application of biomechanical principles can help develop individualized therapy plans, especially when it comes to restoring movement skills after injuries or surgery. The knowledge of biomechanics allows occupational therapists to select appropriate exercises and interventions to improve the functionality and quality of life of their patients.

Bobath Concept/Neurodevelopmental Therapy (NDT)

The Bobath concept, also known as neurodevelopmental therapy (NDT), is a physiotherapy and occupational therapy method that aims to improve the motor functions of people with neurological diseases or damages. It was developed by British physiotherapists Berta and Karel Bobath in the 1940s and has since become an internationally recognised form of therapy.

The Bobath concept is based on the assumption that the nervous system is plastic and can adapt to change. It focuses on promoting normal movement patterns and improving muscle function to maximize functional abilities. The concept is often applied to people with neurological disorders such as stroke, cerebral palsy, trauma to the central nervous system, and other neurological disorders.

Here are some basic principles and features of the Bobath concept:

1. **Individualized treatment:** The Bobath concept emphasizes the need for an individualized and patient-centered approach. Therapists tailor their interventions to the specific needs, abilities, and goals of the individual.
2. **Movement Promotion:** It emphasizes promoting normal movement patterns and improving movement control. Therapists use manual techniques, exercises, and activities to facilitate mobility.
3. **Sensory integration:** The concept also incorporates sensory stimuli into the therapy to support the perception and control of movements. This can include tactile, proprioceptive, and vestibular stimuli.
4. **Analysis of posture and movement:** Therapists carefully analyze posture and movement to identify problematic patterns. The interventions aim to correct faulty patterns and restore normal mobility.
5. **Everyday activities:** The Bobath concept integrates activities relevant to everyday life into the therapy in order to ensure the transferability of the acquired skills to the daily life context.

6. **Teamwork:** An important component of the concept is collaboration in an interdisciplinary team, which can often include physiotherapists, occupational therapists, speech therapists, and other professionals.

The Bobath concept has proven to be an effective method of rehabilitation for people with neurological disorders. However, it is emphasized that the application of the concept should always be adapted to the individual needs and progress of the person.

Body Awareness

Body awareness refers to the ability to receive, interpret and respond to signals from one's own body. It includes various sensory information originating from the sensory organs, muscles, joints, and other tissues. Body awareness plays a crucial role in the way we experience and interact with our own bodies.

Here are some points of body awareness:

1. **Tactile (touch):** The ability to sense touch, pressure, and vibration is crucial for body awareness. This affects not only the skin, but also deeper tissue layers.
2. **Proprioceptive (self-perception):** This is the perception of the position and movement of one's own body in space. Proprioceptive receptors in muscles, tendons, and joints provide the brain with information about body position and movement.
3. **Sense of balance:** The ability to stand upright and move stably depends heavily on the perception of balance. This is controlled by signals from the inner ear, eyes, and proprioceptive receptors.
4. **Pain perception:** The sensation of pain is an important aspect of body awareness. Pain receptors inform the body about possible damage or threats.
5. **Interoception:** This refers to the perception of internal body states such as hunger, thirst, fatigue, and emotional states. It allows us to recognize and respond to our physical needs.

Precise body awareness is important for everyday functioning, coordination of movements, prevention of injuries and adaptation to the environment. Disorders in body perception can occur in various areas, including neurological disorders, developmental disorders, or after injuries. In therapy, especially occupational therapy or physiotherapy, interventions can be used to improve body awareness and address related challenges.

Body imago

The term "body imago" refers to the body image or idea a person has of their own body. It includes subjective perception, evaluation and attitude towards one's own body. The body imago plays an important role in the field of psychology, especially in relation to self-awareness, self-esteem and psychological well-being.

A positive body imago means that a person is content, accepting, or even loving towards their own body. In contrast, a negative body imago can lead to dissatisfaction, self-criticism, and in some cases, mental health problems, such as eating disorders or depression.

Various factors can influence body imago, including cultural norms, social media, personal experiences, upbringing, and individual personality traits. Especially in societies where certain ideals of beauty prevail, the pressure to conform to these ideals can negatively affect the body imago.

Promoting a positive body imago is important for psychological well-being. This can be achieved by developing self-acceptance, realistic self-awareness, and a healthy attitude towards the diversity of body shapes and sizes. Psychological interventions, support groups, and supportive social environments can also help improve body imago, especially if it is compromised by negative self-images.

Body Schema

The body schema refers to the cognitive representation of one's own body in the brain. It is a kind of inner map that allows us to perceive and understand our body and its various parts spatially. The body schema plays a crucial role in the coordination of movements, the perception of touch, and the ability to orient our body in space.

A well-developed body schema allows us to navigate our body without constant visual control. It is the basis of various motor skills and actions, since it helps us understand the position and movement of our limbs without having to look at it all the time.

The body schema develops over the course of childhood through sensory experiences and movement. Healthy body schema development is important for fine motor coordination, balance, and the ability to perform complex tasks.

Disorders in the body schema can lead to various problems, including difficulty with fine motor skills, balance problems, and sensory integration problems. In therapy, especially occupational therapy or physiotherapy, exercises and interventions are often used to improve the body schema and promote motor skills.

It should be noted that the body schema is not static and may evolve throughout life, influenced by experiences, injuries or other life events.

Brain Gym

"Brain Gym" refers to an educational exercise program that aims to promote brain function and support learning. It is based on the idea that certain movements and activities can improve coordination between the brain and the body, which is said to have a positive effect on cognitive abilities, concentration and learning processes.

The Brain Gym program was developed by Paul Dennison, an educational consultant, and his wife, Gail Dennison. It includes a series of simple physical exercises aimed at activating brain functions and improving communication between the cerebral hemispheres. The movements are designed to support specific skills such as reading, writing, attention, and problem-solving.

Some basic principles of the Brain Gym program include:

1. **Exercise:** The idea that physical exercise stimulates brain functions and can promote learning.
2. **Coordination of the cerebral hemispheres:** The assumption that certain exercises can help improve cooperation between the left and right hemispheres of the brain.
3. **Simplicity:** The exercises are simple and can be easily integrated into everyday school life or other learning environments.

Examples of brain gym exercises can be the so-called "cross crawl," in which diagonally opposite extremities (such as the right knee and left hand) are moved in a crossing motion. However, there are various exercises in the Brain Gym program, and it is necessary to know that the scientific evidence for the effectiveness of this approach is limited.

Brain Performance Training

Brain performance training refers to a series of targeted exercises and activities aimed at improving or maintaining cognitive and mental performance. This training is often designed to support people with various forms of cognitive impairment or disorders. Further information on brain power training:

1. **Goals of training:** Brain power training has different goals, depending on the needs and limitations of the individual. These include improving attention, memory, problem-solving skills, concentration, verbal and non-verbal communication, and other cognitive functions.
2. **Target Groups:** Brain performance training is often recommended for people who suffer from cognitive impairment, whether due to neurological conditions such as dementia, stroke, traumatic brain injury, or other causes.
3. **Individual adaptation:** An important principle of brain performance training is the individual adaptation of the exercises to the needs, abilities and progress of the individual. This allows for a targeted and effective intervention.
4. **Cognitive domains:** The training can address various cognitive domains, including:
    - **Memory training:** exercises to strengthen short-term and long-term memory.
    - **Attention training:** Activities that improve the ability to focus and maintain attention.
    - **Problem-solving training:** Exercises that develop the ability to identify, analyze, and find solutions.
    - **Language and communication training:** activities to improve verbal and non-verbal communication skills.
    - **Executive Functional Training:** Exercises that target higher cognitive functions, such as planning, organization, and self-regulation.
5. **Tools and games:** Brain performance training can include various tools and games, including cognitive apps, puzzles,

memory games, word games, and other activities that pose challenges to the brain.
6. **Group or individual training:** Depending on the needs of the individual, brain performance training can be carried out in groups or in an individual setting.
7. **Professionals:** Training is often conducted by professionals, including neuropsychologists, occupational therapists, speech therapists, or other therapists with expertise in cognitive rehabilitation.
8. **Long-term care:** Brain power training can be part of a long-term care plan to promote mental health, slow the progression of cognitive disorders, or improve quality of life.

It should be emphasized that brain performance training should be part of a comprehensive treatment approach that also includes other medical, therapeutic and social interventions, especially in people with neurological diseases or age-related cognitive changes.

Case Conference

A case conference is a joint meeting or discussion between professionals from different disciplines involved in mentoring an individual or a group. In occupational therapy, a case conference can be used to gain comprehensive insights into a patient's needs, progress, and challenges. These conferences promote collaboration and exchange of information between the members of the treatment team. Here are some aspects of a case conference in occupational therapy:

1. **Participant:**
   - Typical participants in an occupational therapy case conference may include occupational therapists, other therapists (e.g., physical therapists, speech therapists), physicians, nurses, social workers, teachers, or other professionals involved in caring for the patient.
2. **Goals:**
   - The goals of a case conference can be manifold. This includes discussing current therapeutic advances, setting or adjusting therapy goals, planning interventions, coordinating care, and identifying barriers to therapy success.
3. **Case presentation:**
   - A member of the treatment team presents the current status of the patient's case. This may include information on diagnosis, therapy history, progress, challenges, and other relevant aspects.
4. **Discussion and exchange of views:**
   - The case conference offers space for the discussion of different perspectives and opinions. Participants will be able to share their expertise and experience to get a comprehensive view of the patient's case.
5. **Collaboration and coordination:**
   - An essential purpose of the case conference is to promote collaboration and coordination between the members of the treatment team. This helps to ensure

that the different interventions are aligned and that care is seamless.
6. **Decision-making:**
   - The case conference can also be used to make joint decisions about the further course of therapy. This may include adjusting therapy goals, introducing new interventions, or referral to other professionals.
7. **Family and patient involvement:**
   - In some cases, the family or the patient himself may also participate in the case conference. This makes it possible to include their perspectives and address their concerns.

The case conference is thus an important mechanism for optimising the quality of care by bringing together expertise from different disciplines to ensure comprehensive and patient-centred care.

Case Management

Case management is a coordinated process of providing comprehensive care and support to people who have complex health, social or legal needs. The aim of case management is to improve the quality of life of those affected by effectively identifying, coordinating and addressing their needs. This approach is applied in various fields, including healthcare, social work, rehabilitation, and other supportive services.

Key features of case management include:

1. **Needs assessment:** A comprehensive assessment identifies a person's individual needs and challenges. This may include medical, social, economic, or legal aspects.
2. **Development of an individual plan:** Based on the needs assessment, a tailor-made plan is created that identifies the necessary services, resources and interventions to address the identified needs.
3. **Coordination of services:** The case manager is responsible for coordinating the various services and resources needed to implement the individual plan. This can include working with various professionals, organizations, and service providers.
4. **Monitoring and adaptation:** The progress of the individual plan is regularly monitored, and the plan is adjusted as needed to ensure it meets the changing needs of the person concerned.
5. **Promoting self-determination:** Case management emphasizes promoting the self-determination and autonomy of the person concerned. The individual plan is developed in close collaboration with the person to take into account their preferences and goals.
6. **Information sharing:** An important aspect is the exchange of relevant information between stakeholders to ensure seamless and efficient care.

Case management is applied in various fields, including health care (health case management), social work (social case management), rehabilitation and nursing. It is especially useful when people with complex and multi-layered needs need support to effectively deal with the different aspects of their lives.

Case study

An occupational therapy case study is a detailed examination of a specific case in which an occupational therapist documents individual observations, interventions, progress, and outcomes. These studies provide deep insight into the application of occupational therapy principles and techniques in the care of an individual patient. Here are some typical elements that might be included in an occupational therapy case study:

1. **Case Description:**
    - An introduction that provides basic information about the patient such as age, gender, medical history, and relevant demographics.
2. **Anamnesis:**
    - A summary of the medical history, including information about the main reasons for presenting to the patient, previous therapy history, and past or current health challenges.
3. **Objectives of occupational therapy:**
    - Clear and measurable objectives to be achieved during occupational therapy interventions. These goals should be based on the individual needs of the patient.
4. **Assessment and findings:**
    - A summary of occupational therapy evaluations and findings, including specific test results and observations, to identify the patient's needs and abilities.
5. **Interventions:**
    - A detailed description of the occupational therapy interventions used to achieve the established objectives. This may include the use of specific activities, exercises, techniques, and tools.
6. **History and progress:**
    - A chronological presentation of the course of therapy, including documented progress or any

challenges. This may also include observations about the patient's responses to the interventions.

7. **Reflection:**
   - A critical reflection on the effectiveness of the interventions applied, possible reasons for success or failure, and adjustments made during the course of therapy.

8. **Outcome and results:**
   - A summary of the results achieved with regard to the objectives set. This may include objective readings, subjective assessments by the patient, and observations by the therapist.

9. **Inference:**
   - A final summary of the case study, including key findings, challenges, successes, and possible recommendations for future interventions.

Case studies not only provide insights into the effectiveness of applied therapy, but also serve as a valuable resource for the advancement of occupational therapy methods and knowledge sharing within the professional community.

Caseload

"Caseload" refers to the number of cases or clients who are cared for by a professional, such as a social worker, therapist, teacher, or healthcare provider. Caseload is an important measure of how many individuals or families a particular professional supports or cares for at the same time.

The size of a caseload can vary significantly, depending on the type of services, the needs of the clients, and the resources of the organization. A large caseload may mean that the professional is responsible for a significant number of people, while a smaller caseload would indicate a smaller number of clients.

Managing the caseload is important to ensure that each person receives appropriate attention and care. Professionals must ensure that they are able to effectively assess each individual's needs, develop individual plans, coordinate resources, and provide appropriate support.

In social work, therapy, nursing, education and other support professions, caseload management plays a central role in ensuring that the quality of care and support is maintained, even when the number of people being cared for is high. A balanced caseload allows professionals to adequately address each individual's needs and provide an effective service.

Cerebral palsy

Cerebral palsy (CP) is a group of permanent movement and posture disorders that can be traced back to a developmental disorder of the brain from early childhood. The impairments arise from abnormal or impaired brain development or function and affect muscle control and coordination of movements.

Here are some key points about cerebral palsy:

1. **Causes:** In most cases, cerebral palsy develops before, during, or shortly after birth. Common causes include prenatal brain damage, birth complications, infections, or genetic factors.
2. **Symptoms:** Symptoms can vary widely, ranging from mild motor impairment to severe disability. The most common symptoms include unusual muscle tension (spasticity or hypotension), coordination problems, balance problems, limited fine motor skills, and limited mobility.
3. **Forms of cerebral palsy:**
   - **Spastic cerebral palsy:** Characterized by increased muscle tension, resulting in stiff movements.
   - **Dyskinetic cerebral palsy:** Characterized by uncontrolled, meandering movements due to impaired muscle control.
   - **Ataxic cerebral palsy:** Characterized by coordination problems and difficulty maintaining balance.
4. **Diagnosis:** Diagnosis is often made in early childhood. Imaging techniques such as MRI can help identify abnormalities in the brain. Developmental history and clinical evaluations also play an important role.
5. **Treatment:** Treatment for cerebral palsy is usually multidisciplinary and includes physical therapy, occupational therapy, speech therapy, and orthopedic interventions where appropriate. Medications can be used to control symptoms such as spasticity. In some cases, orthopedic surgery may be needed to correct deformities or improve mobility.

Caring for people with cerebral palsy requires an individualized approach to promote the best possible quality of life and functionality. Early interventions are crucial to support the development and management of challenges.

Chronic illness

A chronic disease is a long-term medical condition that often lasts for a long period of time and is usually not easily cured. Unlike acute diseases, which have a short-term course, chronic diseases tend to last for a longer period of time or even life. They often require ongoing medical care, self-management, and sometimes lifelong lifestyle adjustments.

Here are some characteristics of chronic diseases:

1. **Long-term course:** Chronic diseases are characterized by a persistent or long-term course, often lasting months or years.
2. **Not easy to cure:** Unlike acute diseases, which are often curable, many chronic diseases cannot be completely cured. The focus is therefore often on managing symptoms and improving quality of life.
3. **Need for ongoing care:** People with chronic illnesses often need regular medical monitoring and care to manage the progression of the disease and prevent complications.
4. **Self-management:** Many chronic diseases require active self-management from sufferers, which may include adherence to medications, lifestyle changes, diet, and exercise.
5. **Multiple causes:** The causes of chronic diseases can be varied, ranging from genetic factors to environmental triggers and lifestyle factors.

Examples of chronic diseases include diabetes, heart disease, rheumatoid arthritis, asthma, chronic obstructive pulmonary disease (COPD), certain forms of cancer, and many others. The treatment of chronic diseases often requires a holistic approach that takes into account various aspects of the individual's life, including physical, psychological, and social aspects.

Chronic polyarthritis/rheumatoid arthritis

Chronic polyarthritis is an outdated term for a specific form of rheumatoid arthritis (RA), an autoimmune disease that primarily affects the joints. Rheumatoid arthritis is a chronic, inflammatory disease in which the body's immune system mistakenly attacks the joints, causing inflammation, pain, swelling, and joint damage.

It should be noted that the term "chronic polyarthritis" is less common today, as it has been replaced by the clearer term "rheumatoid arthritis" to emphasize the specific nature of the condition.

The main features of rheumatoid arthritis (chronic polyarthritis) include:

1. **Symmetrical joint inflammation:** The inflammation often affects joints on both sides of the body, for example, both knees or wrists.
2. **Chronic course:** The disease is chronic and tends to worsen over time if not treated appropriately.
3. **Inflammation and swelling:** The joints are inflamed, causing swelling, pain, and limited mobility.
4. **General symptoms:** In addition to joint symptoms, people with rheumatoid arthritis may also experience general symptoms such as fatigue, weight loss, and muscle weakness.
5. **Autoimmune reaction:** The exact cause of rheumatoid arthritis is not fully understood, but it is an autoimmune disease in which the immune system attacks the body's own joints.

Treatment for rheumatoid arthritis often includes anti-inflammatory drugs, immunosuppressants, and medications designed to slow the progression of the disease. Additionally, physical therapy and lifestyle changes are recommended to improve quality of life and minimize joint damage.

Cocontraction

Cocontraction refers to the simultaneous contraction (tension) of antagonistic muscles or muscle pairs. Antagonistic muscles are muscles that allow opposite movements around a joint. During a movement, one muscle should normally contract, while the antagonistic muscle remains relaxed. However, in cocontraction, both muscles contract at the same time.

This type of muscle activity usually occurs to provide extra stability in a joint, especially when precision and fine motor skills are required. Co-contraction can help protect joints by creating a more stable platform for movement. An example of this is the co-contraction of the muscles around the knee joint to provide stability while walking or standing.

However, cocontraction can also be undesirable in certain situations, especially if it is excessive or inappropriate. In some cases, it can lead to stiffness, restricted movement, or other problems.

In rehabilitation and physiotherapy practice, the control of cocontraction is often considered to improve the ability to move, address muscle imbalances and optimize the function of joints. Targeted exercises and therapeutic approaches can be aimed at improving coordination and control of the muscles and promoting appropriate co-contraction.

Cognitive-Behavioral Therapy

Cognitive-behavioral therapy (CBT) is a widely used form of psychotherapy that aims to treat mental health problems by identifying and modifying negative thought patterns and behaviors. CBT is based on the assumption that thoughts, feelings, and behaviors are interconnected, and that changes in one of these areas can cause change in the others.

Here are some key principles and techniques of Cognitive Behavioral Therapy:

1. **Cognitive restructuring:** CBT aims to identify and change negative thought patterns. This process is called cognitive restructuring. It involves recognizing and reviewing negative or destructive thoughts and replacing them with more realistic and constructive beliefs.
2. **Behavioral activation:** By encouraging positive behaviors and activities, negative emotions and thought patterns can be changed. Behavioral activation aims to promote positive changes in behavior to improve emotional well-being.
3. **Exposure therapy:** This technique is often used for anxiety disorders. It involves the gradual and controlled confrontation with anxiety-inducing situations in order to reduce anxiety.
4. **Development of problem-solving skills:** CBT promotes the development of effective problem-solving skills to better cope with challenges and stressors.
5. **Self-observation and journaling:** Clients are encouraged to observe and record their thoughts and emotions. This can help identify patterns and track changes in thinking and behavior.
6. **Homework:** In CBT, clients are often given homework to apply and practice the skills and techniques they have acquired between sessions.

CBT is successfully used to treat a variety of mental health problems, including depression, anxiety disorders, post-traumatic stress disorder (PTSD), obsessive-compulsive disorder, and many others. This form of therapy is usually time-limited and structured, with clear goals and a focused approach.

Communication aids

Communication aids are tools or strategies designed to support the communication of people who have difficulty speaking or understanding spoken language. These aids are often used for people with various forms of speech or communication disorders, whether due to physical limitations, neurological diseases or developmental disorders. Here are some examples of communication aids:

1. **Image communication systems:**
    - **Pictograms and symbols:** Images or symbols that represent concepts can be used in image communication systems. These can be integrated in the form of printed maps, picture books or electronic devices.
2. **Sign or sign language:**
    - **Sign language:** For people who have difficulty speaking, sign language can be an effective way to express themselves. There are different sign languages around the world, and for some people, an individual form of sign language can also be developed.
3. **Communication Boards:**
    - **Boards with symbols or text:** Communication boards are visual aids on which people can communicate their needs, thoughts, or feelings by pointing to symbols or text.
4. **Electronic Speech Output Devices:**
    - **Tablets or special communication devices:** Electronic speech output devices allow people to communicate by selecting icons, text, or pre-recorded voice messages. Some devices can also be customized to meet individual needs.
5. **Speech therapy:**
    - **Professional support:** Speech therapists can develop individual communication aids and help people with communication disorders improve their language skills.

6. **Visualization aids:**
   - **Visualization of time and tasks:** For people with cognitive challenges, visualization aids, such as schedules or to-do lists with images, can support the communication process.
7. **Supported Communication Software:**
   - **Apps and software:** There are various apps and software programs that are specifically designed for assisted communication. These can be used on tablets or computers and offer a wide range of options for individual customization.
8. **Text-to-speech systems:**
   - **Programs that convert typed text into speech:** These systems can help people who have difficulty speaking to express themselves through typed text.
9. **Communication Partner Training:**
   - **Training for families and caregivers:** People close to the affected person, such as family members, caregivers or teachers, can learn through training how to support and improve communication.

Communication aids should always be adapted to the individual needs and abilities of the person concerned. The selection and application of these aids is often done in collaboration with professionals such as speech therapists, occupational therapists or assisted communication specialists.

Community Integration

Community integration refers to the process and outcome of integrating individuals into the community, especially those who may be impaired by physical, cognitive, or psychosocial challenges. The goal of community integration is to ensure that people are able to actively participate in community life, be socially connected, and improve their quality of life.

Some key aspects of community integration include:

1. **Participation in community life:** This involves participating in social, cultural, religious, and other activities within the community. It's about using individual skills and interests to be an active member of the community.
2. **Self-determination and autonomy:** Community integration promotes the self-determination and autonomy of individuals. This means that people should have the opportunity to make decisions about their lives and pursue their personal goals.
3. **Social relationships:** The development and maintenance of social relationships are crucial elements of community integration. This includes forming friendships, participating in social groups, and interacting with neighbors and community members.
4. **Access to education and employment:** Integration into the community also includes access to education and employment opportunities. This not only creates financial independence, but also contributes to social identity and participation.
5. **Accessibility:** An accessible environment is crucial for community inclusion, especially for people with physical or cognitive impairments. This includes physical accessibility, accessible communication, and the elimination of prejudice and discrimination.

Community integration is relevant in various contexts, including rehabilitation of people with disabilities, mental health care, support for older adults, and much more. Professionals such as occupational therapists, social workers, and other community care professionals often play a role in fostering community integration.

Community-Based Rehabilitation

Community-Based Rehabilitation (CBR) is a concept in health and rehabilitation practice that aims to integrate people with disabilities into their communities and improve their quality of life. CBR emphasizes collaboration between individuals with disabilities, their families, communities, and various professionals to provide comprehensive support and rehabilitation.

Some principles and characteristics of community-based rehabilitation are:

1. **Inclusion and participation:** CBR emphasizes the inclusion of people with disabilities in all aspects of life. It aims to encourage their active participation in social, economic, educational and cultural activities.
2. **Holistic approach:** CBR takes into account not only the physical aspects of the disability, but also social, economic and cultural factors. The approach is holistic and takes into account individual needs, resources and contexts.
3. **Partnership and collaboration:** CBR relies on collaboration between people with disabilities, their families, community members, local organizations, and professionals. A joint effort is sought to understand the needs of the community and provide appropriate support.
4. **Community empowerment:** A key goal of CBR is to strengthen the community to better support people with disabilities and promote their integration. This may include training community members, awareness campaigns, and promoting accessible environments.
5. **Personal responsibility and self-determination:** CBR promotes the self-determination of people with disabilities and encourages them to take an active role in their rehabilitation and participation.

CBR can be implemented in a number of ways, including:

- **Health promotion and rehabilitation:** Through the provision of health services, rehabilitation and support in coping with impairments.
- **Education:** By promoting access to education for people with disabilities and creating inclusive school systems.
- **Employment and economic inclusion:** By supporting the integration of people with disabilities into the labour market and economic activities.

Community-based rehabilitation is particularly relevant in resource-constrained environments and in countries with limited access to specialized health services. It emphasizes the importance of upholding human rights, promoting social justice and breaking down barriers in society.

Concentration

Concentration refers to the ability to focus attention and mental effort on a particular activity, thought, or task. It is a mental state in which attention is focused and focused on what is being done without being disturbed by other stimuli or distractions.

Concentration includes:

1. **Focus: Concentration** involves the ability to focus attention on a particular thing and keep it there. This often requires the suppression of distractions.
2. **Endurance:** Concentration also involves the ability to maintain attention for long periods of time, especially during tasks that require perseverance.
3. **Selective attention:** Concentration often involves the ability to focus on a specific task or information while ignoring other stimuli or information.
4. **Types of concentration:** There are different types of concentration, such as selective concentration (focusing on a specific thing), divided concentration (the ability to handle multiple tasks at once), and sustained concentration (maintaining attention for an extended period of time).

Factors such as fatigue, stress, environment and personal interests can affect the ability to concentrate. Good concentration is essential for effective learning, job performance, problem-solving, and many other mental activities.

Techniques to improve concentration may include meditation, taking breaks during prolonged tasks, organizational strategies, getting enough sleep, and getting regular physical exercise. In case of persistent difficulty with concentration, it may be advisable to seek professional help to identify possible underlying causes and receive appropriate interventions.

Consultation

Counseling refers to a process in which a qualified professional, often referred to as a counselor, works with an individual, group, or organization to provide support, guidance, or advice regarding personal, professional, emotional, or social challenges.

Here are some key aspects in the consulting context:

1. **Confidentiality:** Counselling is often based on a relationship of trust between the counsellor and the client. Confidentiality is crucial to encourage open and honest communication.
2. **Objective:** Counseling focuses on achieving specific goals or overcoming problems. These goals can range from improving emotional well-being to solving concrete challenges in the professional or personal sphere.
3. **Active listening and communication:** The counselor listens carefully and communicates in a way that promotes understanding and empathy. The ability to listen and communicate effectively is crucial to understanding the client's needs.
4. **Empowerment:** Counseling often aims to empower clients to recognize and use their own resources to overcome their challenges. This may include developing skills, building self-confidence, and promoting self-management strategies.
5. **Problem identification and resolution:** The consulting process often involves identifying problems or challenges and collaboratively developing strategies to solve those problems.
6. **Cultural sensitivity:** Counsellors should be culturally sensitive and respect the diversity of clients. This includes taking cultural differences into account and adapting counselling methods to individual needs.

Counseling can take place in a variety of settings, including schools, businesses, healthcare facilities, or private practices. The effectiveness of counseling often depends on the quality of the relationship between counselor and client, the expertise of the counselor, and the client's willingness to cooperate.

Contracture

A contracture refers to the permanent shortening or hardening of muscles, tendons, or connective tissue, resulting in restricted movement in a joint. It can have different causes and can occur in different parts of the body. Contractures can be painful and affect quality of life.

Here are some common types of contractures and their causes:

1. **Muscle contracture:** This refers to a permanent shortening or contraction of a muscle. Causes can be trauma, scarring after injuries, unused muscles after prolonged immobility or neurological disorders.
2. **Tendon contracture:** In tendon contracture, the tendon shortens, which leads to a restriction of joint movement. This can be caused by inflammation, scarring, or degenerative changes in the tendon.
3. **Joint contracture:** This is a limitation of the mobility of a joint due to contractions of the surrounding muscles, tendons or ligaments. Joint contractures can result from prolonged immobility, degenerative joint disease, or scarring after injury.

Prevention and treatment of contractures often include physiotherapy measures, including special stretching exercises, massage, heat or cold therapy, and, if necessary, the use of splints or orthotics to maintain normal joint mobility. In some cases, surgical intervention may be necessary to loosen contracted structures and restore normal mobility. Early intervention is important because untreated contractures can progress and lead to significant functional impairment.

Contracture prophylaxis

Contracture prophylaxis is a preventive measure in medicine and especially in nursing and rehabilitation. A contracture refers to a permanent shortening or stiffening of muscles, tendons, or connective tissue that can lead to limited joint mobility. Contracture prophylaxis aims to prevent or minimize the development of contractures, especially in individuals who are at increased risk for such limitations due to illness, injury, or other conditions.

Here are some strategies that can be used as part of contracture prophylaxis:

1. **Movement exercises and mobilization:** Regular passive and active movement exercises help maintain joint flexibility and stretch muscles. This is especially important for people who are at increased risk due to bedridden or immobility.
2. **Change of position:** By regularly repositioning and changing body position, pressure points can be minimized, which reduces the risk of contractures. This is especially relevant for people who have to remain in the same position for a long time.
3. **Aids and positioning aids:** The use of special pillows, mattresses or positioning aids can help relieve pressure points and support the correct alignment of the joints.
4. **Physical therapy and occupational therapy:** Professionals such as physical therapists and occupational therapists can develop individualized exercise programs that are tailored to the needs of the individual to promote joint mobility.
5. **Skin care:** Good skin care is important to maintain skin integrity and minimize the risk of pressure ulcers, which in turn can favor the appearance of contractures.
6. **Promotion of physical activity:** Promoting activity and movement in everyday life helps to maintain muscle strength and flexibility.

Contracture prophylaxis is particularly relevant in the care of the elderly, long-term patients, people with neurological diseases or after surgical interventions. Individual needs and risk factors should always be taken into account in order to ensure effective and safe prophylaxis.

Coordination

Coordination refers to the body's ability to control and synchronize movements effectively and precisely. Good coordination requires the smooth cooperation of muscles, joints, sensory organs and the central nervous system. Coordination is crucial in various areas of life, including sports, everyday activities, work tasks, and more.

Here are some aspects of coordination:

1. **Fine motor skills:** Fine motor skills refer to precise and coordinated movements of small muscles, especially in the hands and fingers. Examples of fine motor tasks include writing, locking buttons, or operating tools.
2. **Gross motor skills:** Gross motor skills refer to the coordination of larger muscle groups that are responsible for movements such as walking, running, jumping, or lifting heavy objects.
3. **Eye-hand coordination:** This form of coordination refers to effectively combining visual information with hand movements to perform specific tasks. Examples include catching a ball or writing on paper.
4. **Proprioception:** The ability to understand one's body's position and movement in space is crucial for coordination. Proprioceptive signals from muscles, tendons, and joints help ensure accurate perception of body movement.
5. **Bilateral coordination:** This refers to the ability to effectively coordinate movements of both sides of the body. Examples include climbing stairs or keeping your balance on one leg.

Good coordination allows a person to perform tasks efficiently and accurately, whether in sports, work, or daily life. The development of coordination can be promoted through targeted exercises, sports, activities that engage the senses, and a healthy lifestyle. In rehabilitation, coordination is often specifically trained to improve motor function, especially after injuries or illnesses.

Coping Strategies

Coping strategies refer to the behaviors, thought patterns, and emotional approaches that people use to deal with stress, strain, challenges, or difficult life situations. The type of coping strategy chosen can have a significant impact on how well a person can cope with stressors and maintain their mental health.

There are several types of coping strategies, which can be divided into two main categories:

1. **Problem-oriented coping strategies:**
    - **Active coping:** This involves taking actions to tackle and solve the problem head-on. This could be, for example, developing a plan to solve a problem or implementing concrete steps.
    - **Information gathering:** Gathering information to improve understanding of the problem and make informed decisions.
    - **Seek instrumental support:** Seek the help of others, whether emotionally, practically, or financially.
2. **Emotion-oriented coping strategies:**
    - **Acceptance:** Accepting the reality of a situation, even if it is difficult, and adapting one's attitude towards it.
    - **Positive reinterpretation:** The ability to see positive aspects of a stressful situation or to focus on coping and personal growth.
    - **Distraction:** Diverting attention from a stressful thought or situation to provide temporary relief.
    - **Seeking emotional support:** Engaging with others for emotional support.

The choice of coping strategy often depends on the nature of the stressor, individual abilities, personality, and available resources. Effective coping strategies can help reduce stress, maintain mental health, and strengthen the ability to cope with future challenges.

It should be emphasized that not all coping strategies are equally effective, and that healthy coping often involves a combination of problem-oriented and emotion-oriented approaches.

Coping with illness

Disease management refers to the strategies, skills, and adaptations that people use to deal with a condition or health problems. Coping with illness is a dynamic process that includes physical, psychological, and social components. The way people deal with illness can have a significant impact on their quality of life and well-being. Information on coping with the disease:

1. **Acceptance of the disease:**
   - Acknowledging one's own illness and accepting the challenges associated with it are crucial steps in coping with illness.
2. **Information gathering:**
   - Understanding one's illness and available treatment options is important. Informed decisions can help to better manage the disease.
3. **Self-management:**
   - People can learn to actively manage their health by paying attention to a healthy lifestyle, medication intake, physical activity, and other aspects of their health.
4. **Coping:**
   - Develop and apply coping strategies to deal with stress, anxiety, and other emotional challenges. This can include techniques such as relaxation exercises, meditation or psychotherapy.
5. **Social support:**
   - Sharing emotions, experiences, and challenges with others can be an important form of support. Family, friends, and support groups can play a supportive role.
6. **Lifestyle adjustment:**
   - Depending on the type of disease, lifestyle adjustments may be necessary, for example in terms of diet, sleep, stress management and physical activity.
7. **Communication with health workers:**

- Open communication with doctors and other healthcare providers is important. Understanding the course of the disease, treatment options, and possible side effects helps to manage it effectively.

8. **Use your own resources:**
   - Identification and use of one's own strengths and resources to deal with the disease. This can promote the development of self-confidence and resilience.

9. **Long-term perspective:**
   - The ability to take a long-term perspective and set realistic goals is an important part of coping with the disease.

10. **Professional support:**
    - If necessary, seeking professional support from therapists, psychologists, or social workers may be useful to address psychological challenges.

Individual coping strategies may vary depending on the type and severity of the illness, personal resources, and circumstances. It is important to emphasize that coping with illness is an individual process and that people find different ways to deal with their specific health challenges.

Craniosacral Therapy

Craniosacral therapy, also known as craniosacral therapy, is a gentle form of manual therapy that aims to affect the craniosacral system. The craniosacral system includes the structures and fluid rhythm that surround the brain and spinal cord, including the bones of the skull, spine, and membranes that surround the central nervous system.

Some basic principles of craniosacral therapy are:

1. **Rhythm of the craniosacral system:** Therapists believe that there is a subtle rhythm in the craniosacral system that is created by the pulse of the cerebrospinal fluid (the fluid that surrounds the brain and spinal cord). This rhythm is called the craniosacral rhythm.
2. **Energy balancing:** Therapists strive to create a balance in the craniosacral system in order to promote the body's natural self-healing powers.
3. **Gentle touch:** The touches in craniosacral therapy are very light and gentle. The therapist often uses only light pressure or holds certain areas of the body to support the body's self-regulation.
4. **Holistic approach:** The therapy looks at the person as a whole and tries to take into account physical, emotional and energetic aspects.

The areas of application of craniosacral therapy can be varied and include conditions such as headaches, back pain, stress, trauma and emotional distress. It is significant that craniosacral therapy is often considered a complementary method and not a substitute for conventional medical treatments. Scientific evidence on the efficacy of craniosacral therapy is limited, and its use may vary.

It is advisable to consult a qualified therapist before starting any craniosacral therapy and ensure that it is performed by a professional with appropriate training and experience.

Creative Therapy

Design therapy is a method of occupational therapy that aims to use a person's creative expressions to promote their psychological, emotional, and social health. This form of therapy integrates various artistic and craft activities in order to strengthen individual resources and achieve therapeutic goals.

In creative therapy, various media such as art, music, dance, theatre and crafts are used to support the client in expressing themselves, processing emotions, reducing stress and promoting self-awareness. Through creative processes, personal problems, blockages or traumatic experiences can be dealt with in an indirect and metaphorical way.

The therapeutic relationship between the occupational therapist and the client plays an important role in creative therapy. The therapist acts as a supporter and facilitator, guiding the client to explore and use the possibilities of creative expression to achieve personal goals. This may include fostering self-confidence, developing coping strategies, or improving social skills.

Gestalt therapy is often used in a variety of contexts, including working with people with mental illness, neurological disorders, developmental disorders, addictions, or other health problems. Due to the variety of creative media, individual preferences and needs can be taken into account, which expands the applicability of this form of therapy in different settings and for different population groups.

Curative Education

Curative education is a field that deals with the promotion, support and education of people with special needs. The focus is on the individual development, inclusive education and social integration of people with physical, mental, emotional or social impairments. Here are some basic aspects of curative education:

1. **Individualization:** Curative education considers each individual to be unique and takes into account individual needs, strengths and weaknesses. The pedagogical approaches are adapted to the specific requirements and potentials of the individual person.
2. **Inclusion:** A central concern of curative education is the promotion of inclusive educational environments. This means that people with special needs should be integrated into regular educational and social settings as far as possible in order to promote their participation in social life.
3. **Developmental support:** Special education teachers work to promote the holistic development of their protégés. This includes cognitive, social, emotional and motor aspects.
4. **Diagnostics and support planning:** Special education educators often perform diagnostic assessments to understand an individual's specific needs and abilities. Based on this diagnosis, an individual support plan is then created.
5. **Family work:** Cooperation with families and caregivers is an important part of curative education. By involving the family in the educational process, holistic support of the child or young person is made possible.
6. **Communication and interaction:** Special education teachers value positive communication and interaction. This includes the use of appropriate communication tools and methods to ensure that students are reached in the best possible way.
7. **Therapeutic approaches:** Therapeutic approaches can be integrated into curative education, depending on the needs of the person being cared for. These include, for example, speech therapy, occupational therapy, physiotherapy or behavioural therapy.

8. **Social integration:** An important goal of curative education is the promotion of social integration. This includes the development of social skills and participation in social activities.

Special education educators often work in a variety of contexts, including schools, special educational institutions, social institutions, therapy centers, and other organizations. Its work is aimed at creating optimal conditions for the individual development of people with special needs and promoting their integration into society.

Dementia

Dementia disorders are a group of illnesses characterized by loss of cognitive abilities, including memory loss, impaired thinking, judgment, ability to learn, and problems with language. These disorders affect the brain and affect daily activities and the quality of life of those affected.

Some of the most common dementias include:

1. **Alzheimer's disease:** Alzheimer's disease is the most common form of dementia. It is characterized by progressive damage to brain tissue, especially the regions responsible for memory and thinking.
2. **Vascular dementia:** This form of dementia occurs when blood vessels in the brain are blocked or damaged, resulting in a lack of blood supply and oxygen. It can occur as a result of strokes or other vascular problems.
3. **Frontotemporal dementia:** This form primarily affects the frontal and temporal lobes of the brain. It can lead to changes in behavior, personality, language, and social skills.
4. **Lewy body dementia:** Lewy bodies are abnormal accumulations of proteins in the brain. This form of dementia can cause hallucinations, Parkinson's-like symptoms, and fluctuations in thinking.
5. **Mixed dementia:** Some people may experience symptoms of several types of dementia at the same time, this is called mixed dementia. A common combination is Alzheimer's disease and vascular dementia.

The exact causes of dementia are complex and can vary from disease to disease. Genetic factors, environmental factors, inflammation in the brain, and vascular disease may play a role.

There is no cure for dementia, but early diagnosis and a comprehensive approach to care and support can improve the quality of life of those affected. Drug treatments, cognitive therapy, nursing support, and adaptation of the environment can all be part of a comprehensive care plan.

Caring for people with dementia often requires close collaboration between healthcare providers, caregivers, family members, and other caregivers. Both the physical and emotional needs of those affected should be taken into account.

Diabetes management

Diabetes management refers to the measures and strategies people with diabetes take to control their blood sugar levels, promote healthy lifestyle habits, and minimize the risk of diabetes complications. Here are some features of diabetes management:

1. **Blood glucose monitoring:** Regular monitoring of blood glucose levels is crucial to determine how food, physical activity, medications, and other factors affect blood sugar levels.
2. **Nutritional management:** A balanced and healthy diet plays a central role in diabetes management. Controlling carbohydrates, fat, and protein, as well as paying attention to portion sizes, can help regulate blood sugar levels.
3. **Drug therapy:** Depending on the type of diabetes (type 1 diabetes, type 2 diabetes, or other forms), medications such as insulin, oral antidiabetic drugs, or other medications may be necessary. Adherence to medication schedules prescribed by the doctor is important.
4. **Physical activity:** Regular physical activity helps lower blood sugar levels, control body weight, and improve insulin sensitivity. It is important to incorporate physical activity into your daily lifestyle.
5. **Weight management:** Maintaining a healthy weight or losing weight when you are overweight can improve blood sugar regulation and reduce the risk of complications.
6. **Blood pressure and cholesterol management:** People with diabetes have an increased risk of cardiovascular disease. Controlling blood pressure and cholesterol levels is therefore important to minimize the risk of cardiovascular complications.
7. **Training and self-management:** Training programs help people with diabetes understand their condition and develop the skills needed to live with it successfully. This may include training on blood glucose monitoring, nutritional counseling, medication management, and lifestyle adjustments.

8. **Regular medical care:** Regular visits to the doctor are crucial to monitor health status, make adjustments to the treatment plan, and detect potential complications early.

Diabetes management requires an individualized approach, as each person's needs are different. A team of doctors, diabetes consultants, dietitians, nurses, and other professionals can help develop a customized plan and provide the support needed for successful diabetes management.

Diagnostics

Diagnostics refers to the process of identifying, evaluating, and classifying diseases, conditions, or problems based on signs, symptoms, and various methods of examination. The goal of diagnostics is to make an accurate assessment of a patient's health status in order to plan an appropriate treatment or intervention. Diagnostics is a central part of medical practice and includes various characteristics:

1. **Medical history:** The doctor collects information about the patient's medical history, including symptoms, duration of discomfort, family history, previous illnesses, and medication use.
2. **Physical exam:** The doctor will perform a thorough exam to identify physical signs and symptoms that could indicate a specific medical condition.
3. **Laboratory tests:** Blood tests, urine tests, imaging (such as X-rays, CT scans, or MRIs), and other laboratory procedures may be performed to obtain objective information about health status.
4. **Functional tests:** Depending on the suspicion of certain diseases, specific functional tests can be performed. Examples include pulmonary function tests, cardiovascular tests, or neurological examinations.
5. **Psychological tests:** In psychology, various tests can be used to assess cognitive function, personality traits, or mental health conditions.
6. **Imaging tests:** Radiological examinations, such as CT, MRI, or ultrasound, can provide detailed images of the inside of the body and help make a diagnosis.
7. **Biopsy:** In some cases, a tissue sample (biopsy) may be taken and examined under a microscope to diagnose certain conditions, especially cancer.
8. **Genetic testing:** If genetic diseases are suspected, genetic testing can be done to identify abnormalities in the genetic material.

Diagnosis can be a one-time affair or change over time, especially as new information or test results become available. An accurate diagnosis forms the basis for developing an appropriate treatment plan and allows healthcare providers to provide the best possible care.

Differential diagnosis

Differential diagnosis refers to the process by which a doctor or medical professional differentiates between different diseases or conditions in order to identify the cause of symptoms. This diagnostic approach helps to consider different possibilities and ultimately make an accurate diagnosis. Differential diagnosis plays a crucial role in medical practice and helps to avoid misdiagnosis.

Here are some key points of differential diagnosis:

1. **Medical history (patient history):** The doctor collects information about the patient's symptoms, medical history, existing medical conditions, medication use, lifestyle, and other relevant factors.
2. **Physical exam:** A thorough physical exam is done to identify signs or symptoms that could indicate certain medical conditions.
3. **Laboratory and imaging tests:** Blood tests, imaging procedures such as X-rays, CT or MRI scans, and other specialized tests may be performed to obtain additional information.
4. **Exclusion diagnoses:** The doctor gradually excludes certain diagnoses based on the information collected and the results of examinations.
5. **Prioritization of diagnoses:** Based on the data collected, the physician prioritizes the most likely diagnoses, taking into account the severity of symptoms, the relevance of risk factors, and other clinical information.
6. **Further examinations:** If necessary, additional specialized examinations or consultations with specialists may be carried out to refine the diagnosis.
7. **Response to therapy:** In some cases, the doctor may make a preliminary diagnosis and prescribe therapeutic intervention. The patient's response to this intervention may provide further clues to the underlying cause.

Differential diagnosis is especially important in complex medical situations where multiple medical conditions can cause similar symptoms. A careful and systematic approach is crucial to make an accurate diagnosis and plan the best possible treatment. Collaboration between doctors, specialists and other healthcare providers plays an important role in this.

Diplegia

Diplegia refers to a form of paralysis in which two symmetrical parts of the body are affected. Paralysis usually occurs due to damage or disruption in the central nervous system. These can impair the development and function of nerve cells and lead to restricted movement.

The most common form of diplegia is spastic diplegia, which is often associated with a form of cerebral palsy (CP). In spastic diplegia, the legs are usually more affected than the arms. Symptoms may include spasticity (increased muscle tone), stiffness, coordination problems, and gait problems. The causes of diplegia can be varied and can be congenital or acquired. Possible causes include:

1. **Periventricular leukomalacia (PVL):** Damage to the white tissue of the brain near the ventricles, common in premature infants.
2. **Hypoxic ischemic encephalopathy (HIE):** Damage to the brain due to lack of oxygen or insufficient blood supply during childbirth or the first hours of life.
3. **Cerebral dysgenesis:** developmental disorders of the brain that can be caused by genetic or environmental factors.
4. **Infections or inflammation:** Infections in the central nervous system can lead to damage.
5. **Traumatic brain injury:** Injuries to the brain can lead to paralysis.

Treatment for diplegia depends on the underlying cause and the individual needs of the patient. Physical therapy, occupational therapy, muscle relaxation medications, and in some cases, surgery may be part of the treatment plan. Early intervention and comprehensive care are often critical to improving quality of life and supporting the development of children with diplegia.

Down syndrome/trisomy 21

Down syndrome, also known as trisomy 21, is a genetic condition caused by the presence of an extra copy of chromosome 21. People with Down syndrome therefore have a total of three copies of chromosome 21 instead of the usual two. This additional genetic information can lead to various physical and mental developmental traits.

Characteristic features of Down syndrome may include:

1. **Delayed development:** Children with Down syndrome may develop more slowly in their motor, cognitive, and language skills than children without this genetic change.
2. **Characteristic facial features:** These include flattened features, slanted eyes, a flat bridge over the nose, and a tongue that may stick out a bit.
3. **Low muscle tone:** Many people with Down syndrome have low muscle tone, which can lead to loose flexibility.
4. **Heart defects:** Heart defects are more common in people with Down syndrome.
5. **Increased risk of certain health problems:** These include thyroid problems, hearing problems, vision problems, and an increased risk of infections.
6. **Intellectual impairments:** People with Down syndrome often have an intellectual disability that can range from mild to moderate.

It is important to emphasize that people with Down syndrome have individual abilities, strengths, and weaknesses. The intensity of the impairments can vary significantly from person to person.

The cause of the occurrence of Down syndrome is largely genetic and occurs randomly. The risk increases with the age of the mother. There are several methods of prenatal diagnosis to identify Down syndrome during pregnancy, such as non-invasive prenatal testing (NIPT) and more invasive methods such as amniocentesis or chorionic villus sampling.

Early intervention, supportive therapies, inclusive education, and a positive, supportive environment can improve the quality of life and skills of people with Down syndrome. With appropriate support, many people with Down syndrome can lead a self-determined and fulfilling lifestyle.

Dysarthria

Dysarthria is a motor speech disorder caused by difficulty controlling or coordinating the muscles involved in speech formation. This disorder leads to impairments in the articulation, intonation, volume and rhythm of spoken language. Dysarthria can result from damage to the central or peripheral nervous system that controls the muscles for speech.

Causes of dysarthria may include:

1. **Stroke:** A stroke that affects the brain regions responsible for language production can lead to dysarthria.
2. **Traumatic brain injury:** Injuries to the brain from accidents, falls, or blows can cause dysarthria.
3. **Neurodegenerative diseases:** Diseases such as amyotrophic lateral sclerosis (ALS), Parkinson's disease, Huntington's disease, and certain forms of dementia can cause dysarthria.
4. **Inflammatory diseases:** Autoimmune diseases or inflammatory processes that affect the nervous system can trigger dysarthria.
5. **Brain tumors:** Tumors in the brain can affect nerve pathways and lead to dysarthria.

The symptoms of dysarthria can vary depending on the cause and the nerves involved. The most common signs include:

1. **Unclear pronunciation:** Difficulty forming words and sounds.
2. **Altered pitch and intonation:** Speech melody may be impaired, which can lead to monotonous speech or unusual pitches.
3. **Slower rate of speech:** The ability to pronounce words quickly and fluently may be impaired.
4. **Difficulty swallowing:** Dysarthria can also affect the muscles in the mouth and throat, which can lead to swallowing problems.
5. **Fatigue:** Talking can be exhausting, and people with dysarthria may get tired more quickly.

Treatment for dysarthria depends on the underlying cause and the severity of symptoms. Speech therapy is often an essential part of treatment to improve speech skills and facilitate communication. In some cases, drug or surgical approaches may also be considered. The exact treatment is determined in consultation with a specialist and a speech therapist.

Dyscalculia

Dyscalculia is a specific learning disorder that involves difficulty developing math skills. People with dyscalculia, despite having normal intelligence, have difficulty understanding mathematical concepts, learning mathematical facts, and performing mathematical operations. These difficulties can extend to various areas of mathematics, including arithmetic, algebra, geometry, and other mathematical disciplines.

Symptoms of dyscalculia may include:

1. **Difficulty with basic math operations:** Adding, subtracting, multiplying, and dividing numbers can be problematic.
2. **Problems in understanding mathematical concepts:** Difficulty grasping mathematical concepts and relationships.
3. **Problems remembering math facts:** Difficulty quickly retrieving numerical facts, such as multiplication tables.
4. **Difficulty in applying mathematical strategies: Problems** in applying specific mathematical strategies or approaches.
5. **Difficulty solving math problems: Problems** in analyzing and solving math problems.

Dyscalculia can have various causes, including genetic factors, neurological differences, or environmental factors. It is important to note that dyscalculia is not due to a lack of interest or effort. It is a neurological condition that causes specific difficulties in mathematical learning.

The diagnosis of dyscalculia is usually made by specialized professionals such as psychologists or educators who specialize in learning difficulties. A comprehensive assessment can be done to identify the individual's mathematical abilities and weaknesses.

The intervention can take various forms and often includes:

1. **Individual learning support:** Tailor-made learning programs tailored to the specific needs of the person.
2. **Use of visual aids:** Use of visual representations, manipulative materials, and other visual aids to illustrate mathematical concepts.
3. **Training of mathematical strategies:** Development and training of specific mathematical strategies to solve mathematical problems.
4. **Early intervention:** Early identification of difficulties and appropriate interventions can help minimize the impact of dyscalculia.

The support of teachers, parents, and professionals is critical to helping people with dyscalculia develop their math skills and function successfully in school and everyday settings.

Dyslexia

Dyslexia is a specific learning disorder that causes difficulty in learning and applying reading skills. People with dyslexia have difficulty reading, spelling, and sometimes writing, despite normal intelligence and adequate academic efforts. Dyslexia affects the ability to identify letters and words, phonological processing (recognizing and manipulating sounds), and word recognition.

Symptoms of dyslexia may include:

1. **Difficulty reading words:** People with dyslexia may have difficulty recognizing words quickly and accurately.
2. **Difficulty decoding:** Difficulty deciphering words into their phonetic components may occur.
3. **Spelling issues:** Spelling errors are common, and it can be difficult to remember the correct spelling of words.
4. **Slow reading pace:** Reading can be more time-consuming than with peers without dyslexia.
5. **Difficulty understanding what is being read:** The connection between reading text and understanding the content may be compromised.

Dyslexia is a neurological disorder that is genetic and affects the structure and function of the brain. It concerns the way the brain processes characters and sounds, especially in relation to the processing of phonological information. Dyslexia is not a consequence of lack of intelligence or poor academic efforts.

The diagnosis of dyslexia is usually made by specialized professionals, such as psychologists or educators who specialize in learning disabilities. A comprehensive assessment can be performed to identify the specific reading and spelling difficulties of the affected person.

Intervention for dyslexia can take various forms and often includes:

1. **Intensive reading and spelling support:** Special learning programs tailored to the individual needs of the person.
2. **Phonological Awareness Training: Exercises** to improve the ability to identify, manipulate, and understand sounds.
3. **Multisensory learning:** The use of different senses, such as sight, hearing, and touch, to promote learning.
4. **Early intervention:** Early identification of difficulties and appropriate interventions can help minimize the impact of dyslexia.

With proper support and intervention, people with dyslexia can become successful readers and learners. Early identification and a positive, supportive environment are critical to dealing with the challenges associated with this learning disorder.

Dysphasia

Dysphasia refers to a speech disorder that causes difficulty in developing and using language. Unlike dyslexia, which focuses on reading and writing, dysphasia specifically affects oral language. People with dysphasia may have difficulty pronouncing words, understanding language, forming grammatically correct sentences, and finding appropriate words.

It is important to explain that dysphasia cannot be explained by sensory or motor impairments, hearing loss, or a general delay in mental development. Dysphasia is a distinct language disorder that is often detected in childhood.

Symptoms of dysphasia may include:

1. **Difficulty understanding language:** Difficulty understanding spoken or written words and phrases.
2. **Limited expressiveness:** Difficulty formulating sentences and expressing thoughts.
3. **Pronunciation problems:** Unclear pronunciation of words and difficulty forming sounds.
4. **Impaired grammar:** Difficulty in applying grammatical rules when speaking.
5. **Vocabulary deficits:** Limited vocabulary and difficulty finding appropriate words.

The causes of dysphasia can be manifold and include genetic factors, neurological diseases or brain injuries. Early intervention is crucial to minimize the effects of dysphasia and promote language skills.

Treatment for dysphasia usually involves speech therapy, in which specially trained professionals work with the individual on various language skills. This therapy can aim to improve phonological awareness, promote expressiveness, develop grammar, and improve understanding of language.

It is important to identify dysphasia early and provide individualized interventions to ensure the best opportunities for language development and participation in social life.

Dyspraxia

Dyspraxia, also known as developmental or coordination disorder, refers to difficulty planning and executing purposeful movements. People with dyspraxia may have difficulty with everyday activities that require precise coordination of muscles and movements. These difficulties can affect various areas, including motor skills, fine motor skills, gross motor skills, and hand-eye coordination.

Symptoms of dyspraxia may include:

1. **Fine motor difficulties:** Problems writing, drawing, cutting, buttoning, or other activities that require precise hand movements.
2. **Gross motor difficulties:** Challenges in catching, throwing, balancing, or other gross motor activities.
3. **Difficulty orienting space:** Difficulty understanding space and distances, which can lead to frequent tripping or bumping.
4. **Coordination problems:** Difficulty coordinating movements, especially if they are sequential or complex.
5. **Hand-eye coordination problems:** Difficulty hitting targets accurately with the hands, especially during fast or unpredictable movements.
6. **Difficulty adapting to new tasks:** People with dyspraxia may have difficulty adapting quickly to new or unfamiliar tasks.

The causes of dyspraxia are not fully understood, but it is thought that genetic factors, developmental delays, or neurological differences may play a role. It is important to note that dyspraxia is not due to a lack of intelligence or effort.

Intervention for dyspraxia can take various forms and often includes:

1. **Occupational therapy:** Specially trained occupational therapists can work with individuals to improve motor skills and develop strategies to overcome challenges.

2. **Physical therapy:** For gross motor challenges, physical therapy can be supportive to improve coordination and strength.
3. **Speech therapy:** In some cases, speech therapy may be indicated to improve oral and verbal coordination.
4. **Adaptations and supports:** Individual adjustments may be required in school or work settings to meet the needs of individuals with dyspraxia.

Early identification and intervention are crucial to help people with dyspraxia develop their motor skills and function successfully in school, work, and everyday activities.

Early Intervention

Early intervention refers to measures and interventions aimed at supporting children's development in the earliest years of life and identifying and addressing potential developmental delays or impairments at an early stage. The focus is on offering children optimal development opportunities and developing their individual potential. Early intervention can be applied in a variety of areas, including physical, cognitive, linguistic, social, and emotional development. Here are some characteristics of early intervention:

1. **Early detection and diagnosis:**
   - Early intervention often begins with identifying developmental delays or potential challenges. This can be done through regular developmental observations, screenings, and early childhood examinations.
2. **Interdisciplinary cooperation:**
   - Early intervention often involves the collaboration of various professionals, including doctors, occupational therapists, speech therapists, psychologists, and educators. Interdisciplinary collaboration enables comprehensive assessment and intervention.
3. **Family-centered approach:**
   - Family involvement is a key aspect of early intervention. Parents and family members are involved in the process and encouraged to actively participate in their child's development. You will receive information, support and resources.
4. **Developmental activities:**
   - Early intervention includes targeted activities and games aimed at promoting physical, cognitive, linguistic and social development. This can include playful learning, movement therapy, language development, and other approaches.
5. **Individualized interventions:**
   - Every child is unique, and therefore early intervention measures are tailored to the child's individual needs,

abilities and interests. Interventions can be both preventive and reactive.

6. **Inclusion:**
   - Early intervention emphasizes inclusive practices to ensure that all children, regardless of abilities or limitations, receive the necessary support to support their development.

7. **Transitions:**
   - Early intervention can support the child's transition to kindergarten or other education and care facilities. This may also include coordination with schools and other institutions.

8. **Holistic approach:**
   - Early intervention takes a holistic view of a child's development, taking into account various dimensions, including physical health, social-emotional development, cognitive abilities, and communication skills.

Early intervention plays a crucial role in maximising children's potential and reducing potential developmental delays. Early and appropriate support can have a positive impact on a child's entire life.

Early rehabilitation

Early rehabilitation refers to specialized and comprehensive rehabilitation measures that are initiated early after a serious illness, injury or operation. The aim of early rehabilitation is to improve the functional abilities and quality of life of patients by starting as early as possible after the onset of the health event. This form of rehabilitation is especially important for patients who require intensive medical care due to serious illnesses or injuries.

Further information on early rehabilitation:

1. **Time of onset:**
   - Early rehabilitation often begins in the hospital while the patient is still under medical supervision. The early start allows for rapid intervention and promotes the best possible results.
2. **Interdisciplinary team:**
   - Early rehabilitation involves an interdisciplinary team of professionals, including doctors, physiotherapists, occupational therapists, speech therapists, nurses and social workers. The collaboration of these professionals aims to provide comprehensive support.
3. **Functional Recovery:**
   - The focus is on restoring functional abilities, including mobility, self-care, and cognitive function. This can be done through targeted exercises, therapeutic interventions, and functional activities.
4. **Adaptation to individual needs:**
   - Early rehabilitation is strongly tailored to the individual needs of the patient. This includes taking into account the specific diagnosis, physical and cognitive abilities, and personal goals and preferences.
5. **Patient and family involvement:**
   - The involvement of patients and their relatives is an important aspect of early rehabilitation. The aim is to

promote the independence of patients and to involve their relatives in the rehabilitation process.
6. **Continuity of care:**
    - Early rehabilitation strives for a seamless handover of patient care to downstream rehabilitation phases or the transition to home. Continuous care and support are crucial for the success of rehabilitation.
7. **Psychosocial support:**
    - In addition to physical recovery, early rehabilitation also takes into account psychosocial aspects. This may include counseling, psychological support, and coping with emotional challenges.
8. **Prevention of complications:**
    - Early rehabilitation aims to prevent complications that may arise due to being bedridden or limited mobility. This includes the prevention of pressure ulcers, breathing problems, and muscle breakdown.

Early rehabilitation is particularly relevant for patients with stroke, traumatic injury, major surgery, or other acute medical events. Early initiation of rehabilitative interventions helps to maximize rehabilitation effects and improve patients' quality of life.

Endurance training

Endurance exercise, also known as aerobic exercise or cardiovascular exercise, is a form of physical activity that aims to improve heart and lung function and increase endurance. It is a form of exercise in which larger muscle groups are active at a moderate intensity for a longer period of time. The main goal is to increase the body's ability to produce and maintain energy for an extended period of time.

Here are some common forms of endurance training:

1. **Running/jogging:** Running or jogging outdoors or on a treadmill is a popular method for endurance training.
2. **Cycling:** Both outdoor cycling and indoor cycling are effective ways to improve cardiovascular endurance.
3. **Swimming:** Swimming is an endurance training that is easy on the joints and is particularly suitable for people with joint problems.
4. **Walking:** Brisk walking over long distances can be an effective form of endurance training.
5. **Rowing:** Rowing, whether on the water or on a rowing ergometer, is a great way to activate many muscles and promote endurance.
6. **Dancing:** Dance activities, whether it's Zumba, aerobics, or other forms of dance, offer not only endurance training, but also fun and variety.

The benefits of endurance training include improved cardiovascular health, increased endurance, increased energy, improved mood, and promoting weight loss or control.

Environmental Modification

Environmental modification refers to targeted changes in a person's physical or social environment to improve their functionality, safety, or quality of life. These adjustments can be made in a variety of areas, including homes, workplaces, schools, and public facilities. The purpose of environmental modification is to take into account the individual needs of people with different abilities or limitations and to promote their participation in social life.

Here are some examples of environmental modifications:

1. **Barrier-free access:** The construction of ramps, elevators or other barrier-free access points in buildings can make it easier for people with mobility impairments to access rooms.
2. **Adaptations in the living area:** This may include the installation of grab bars, non-slip floors, height-adjustable countertops, or other customizations to promote independence for people with physical limitations.
3. **Lighting and contrast**: Adjusting lighting and color contrasts indoors can help people with visual impairments move more safely and efficiently.
4. **Technological aids:** The integration of technologies such as speech recognition, communication devices, or smart home appliances can help people with cognitive or motor impairments.
5. **Workplace adaptations:** This includes ergonomic furniture, flexible working hours, screen readers, and other customizations to make the workplace more accessible to people with different needs.
6. **Noise control measures:** Reducing noise or creating quiet work or living areas can benefit people with sensory sensitivities.
7. **Information and guidance:** Providing clear information, for example through legible signage or tactile guidance systems, can make it easier for people with visual or cognitive impairments to find their way around.

Environmental modifications are often carried out in collaboration with professionals such as occupational therapists, architects, social workers, or other experts to ensure that the adaptations meet individual needs and requirements. Through such modifications, people with different abilities can function better in their environment and lead a more self-determined life.

Equestrian Therapy/Hippotherapy/Equine-Assisted Therapy (EAT)

Equestrian therapy, also known as hippotherapy, equine assisted therapy, or equine-assisted therapy, is a form of therapy that involves horses in the treatment process to promote the physical, emotional, cognitive, and social development of people. The term "hippotherapy" is derived from the Greek words "hippos" (horse) and "therapeia" (therapy). Further information on equestrian therapy:

1. **Objectives and applications:**
    - Equestrian therapy is used for a variety of purposes, including improving motor skills, balance and coordination skills, emotional regulation, attention, social skills, and quality of life. It is often used for people with physical, cognitive, or emotional impairments.
2. **Integration of the horse:**
    - The horse plays a central role in equestrian therapy. The horse's natural movements, especially the gait of the walk, have a beneficial effect on the rider's musculature and sensory perception.
3. **Movement of the horse:**
    - The three-dimensional, rhythmic movement of the horse simulates human walking movements and has a positive effect on the development and strengthening of muscles, balance and coordination.
4. **Customization:**
    - The riding therapy is individually adapted to the needs of each participant. The type and intensity of exercises may vary depending on the goals of the therapy and the abilities of the individual.
5. **Therapeutic support:**
    - A specially trained therapist (often a physiotherapist, occupational therapist or psychologist) leads the riding therapy sessions. The therapist adjusts the exercises and monitors the participant's progress.

6. **Promoting social interaction:**
    - Interacting with the horse also promotes social skills and emotional bonding. The need to interact with the horse creates opportunities for communication, collaboration, and teamwork.
7. **Confidence:**
    - The relationship between the rider and the horse fosters trust and emotional bonding. The experience of interacting with a large animal can boost self-confidence and provide a sense of control.
8. **Physical Benefits:**
    - The movement of the horse helps in strengthening the core muscles, improving posture, increasing flexibility and promoting proprioceptive stimuli.
9. **Cognitive stimuli:**
    - Participating in equestrian therapy can also promote cognitive skills such as attention, concentration, and problem-solving.
10. **Leisure and quality of life:**
    - Apart from the therapeutic benefits, equine therapy offers participants the opportunity to participate in recreational activities and improve quality of life.

Equestrian therapy has proven to be an effective complement to traditional forms of therapy and is used in various therapeutic contexts to improve the quality of life of people with different needs.

Equilibrium

Balance refers to the body's ability to remain stable and maintain its position, whether at rest or during movement. Balance is a complex process that is influenced by various factors, including the vestibular system in the inner ear, visual perception, and proprioceptive receptors in muscles and joints.

There are two main types of equilibrium:

1. **Static equilibrium:** This refers to the ability to maintain a stable position at rest without moving. An example of this is standing on one leg.
2. **Dynamic balance:** This refers to the ability to maintain balance during movement, whether it's walking, running, or other activities. Dynamic balance requires the ability to respond to changes in body position.

The interplay between the vestibular system, visual perception and proprioceptive information allows the brain to constantly receive information about the position of the body in space and respond appropriately. Problems in one of these systems or an impairment of the muscles can affect balance.

Various factors can affect balance, including age, neurological disorders, musculoskeletal problems, dizziness, and other health conditions.

Promoting balance is important to prevent falls and injuries. This can be achieved through various exercises and activities specifically aimed at improving balance skills. These include balance exercises, proprioceptive training, coordinative exercises, and specific sports or activities such as yoga or tai chi.

In rehabilitation after injuries or in the case of certain illnesses, targeted therapy, for example by physiotherapists or occupational therapists, may be necessary to restore balance and improve mobility.

Evaluation

"Evaluation" in the context of occupational therapy refers to the process of systematically assessing people's abilities, skills, activities, and participation. Occupational therapy uses different assessment tools and methods to understand a patient's current condition, identify specific goals, and monitor the course of therapy. Here are some characteristics of evaluation in occupational therapy:

1. **Anamnesis and findings:**
    - Occupational therapists perform a comprehensive medical history to gather information about the patient's medical history, life circumstances, and individual goals.
    - The assessment includes physical, cognitive, psychosocial and sensory assessment.
2. **Standardized Tests and Measurement Instruments:**
    - Occupational therapists use standardized tests and measurement instruments to quantify and compare specific skills. This may include the assessment of fine motor skills, gross motor skills, cognitive skills, and other aspects.
    - Examples of such instruments are the "Jebsen-Taylor Hand Function Test" for hand function or the "COPM" (Canadian Occupational Performance Measure) for assessing independence in activities of daily living.
3. **Observation:**
    - Direct observation of the patient during specific activities can provide important information about their abilities and challenges.
    - Occupational therapists can analyze the patient's interactions with their environment to identify potential obstacles or opportunities for support.
4. **Talks and interviews:**
    - Informal conversations and structured interviews allow occupational therapists to learn more about the patient's perspective on their own abilities and the difficulties they are experiencing.

- This encourages a client-centered approach to therapy.
5. **Functional Assessment:**
    - Evaluation in occupational therapy often focuses on a patient's functional abilities, especially with regard to activities of daily living (ADLs) and instrumental activities of daily living (IADLs).
6. **Objective:**
    - Based on the results of the evaluation, occupational therapists work with the patient to set clear, achievable goals for therapy.
    - The goals are formulated specifically for the needs and desires of the individual.

Evaluation is a continuous process in occupational therapy, as it allows therapists to tailor the therapy plan and ensure that interventions are tailored to the patient's individual needs.

Executive Functions

Executive functions are cognitive processes in the brain that are responsible for self-regulation, planning, organizing, initiating, and controlling behavior and thinking. These functions play a crucial role in carrying out day-to-day activities and achieving long-term goals. The executive functions make it possible to process information, act in a goal-oriented manner, and respond appropriately to various requirements. Executive functions include:

1. **Working Memory:**
    - Working memory refers to the ability to retain information for short periods of time and work with it at the same time. It is important for tasks such as following instructions, solving problems, and planning activities.
2. **Inhibition:**
    - Inhibition refers to the ability to suppress impulsive reactions and make deliberate decisions instead. It's important to avoid distractions and focus on the most important tasks.
3. **Flexibility:**
    - Flexibility refers to the ability to adapt to changing conditions, change plans, and find different approaches to a task. It is crucial for adaptability in daily life.
4. **Initiation:**
    - Initiation refers to the ability to begin an action or set a process in motion. Difficulties in this area can lead to procrastination.
5. **Planning and organization:**
    - Planning and organization involve the ability to plan steps to achieve a goal and use resources efficiently. Difficulties in this area can lead to problems in structuring tasks.

6. **Self-control:**
    - Self-control refers to the ability to regulate emotions, prevent impulsive actions, and prioritize long-term goals over short-term gratifications.
7. **Metacognition:**
    - Metacognition refers to the awareness of one's own thought processes and the ability to monitor and regulate them. This is important for effective problem-solving and strategic thinking.
8. **Social Cognition:**
    - Social cognition refers to the ability to understand social situations, navigate interpersonal relationships, and respond appropriately to social cues.

Difficulties in executive functions can occur with various conditions, including ADHD, autism, stroke, or other neurological disorders. Occupational therapists can assist in the development and improvement of these functions through targeted interventions to promote independence and quality of life.

Expressive Therapy

Expression therapy refers to a variety of therapeutic approaches that use creative expression, such as art, music, dance, drama, or writing, to manage and process emotional, psychological, or physical challenges. This form of therapy allows people to express their feelings, thoughts, and experiences in a non-verbal way.

Here are some of the main forms of expression therapy:

1. **Art therapy:** This approach uses artistic mediums such as painting, drawing, pottery, or crafts to encourage individual expression. The resulting artworks serve as a means of communication and self-knowledge.
2. **Music therapy:** Music is used as a tool to promote emotional expression, reduce stress, and achieve therapeutic goals. This may include singing, playing an instrument, or listening to music.
3. **Dance and Movement Therapy:** Through the use of movement and dance, physical expressions are used to explore and process psychological and emotional states.
4. **Drama Therapy:** This uses dramatic elements such as role-playing, improvisation and theatre exercises to shed light on personal challenges and explore alternative perspectives.
5. **Writing therapy (also called bibliotherapy):** Writing is used as a therapeutic tool to record and reflect on thoughts, feelings, or experiences. Keeping a diary, poetry or writing stories are possible forms.

Expression therapy is based on the assumption that creative activities provide a unique access to inner emotions and experiences, and that the creative process itself can have healing properties. A trained therapist accompanies the individual in choosing their form of expression and promoting the therapeutic process.

This form of therapy is used in various settings, including mental health practices, schools, hospitals, and rehabilitation centers, to help people cope with stress, trauma, anxiety, depression, and other challenges.

Fine motor skills

Fine motor skills refers to the precise movements of small muscles that allow a person to perform targeted and controlled actions. These movements mainly affect the hands, fingers and wrists. Developing and maintaining well-developed fine motor skills are crucial for performing everyday activities, especially for tasks that require high precision. Fine motor skills include, among other things:

1. **Grab:**
   - Grasping refers to the ability to hold and manipulate objects with one's hands. There are several gripping techniques, including the three-point grip (thumb and the first two fingers), the tweezer grip (thumb and one of the fingers), and the lateral grip (thumb on the side of the fingers).
2. **Hand-eye coordination:**
   - The ability to coordinate vision with hand movements is crucial. This allows precise actions, such as writing, drawing or operating small objects.
3. **Dexterity:**
   - Dexterity involves the ability to move and control individual fingers independently. This is especially important for fine activities, such as buttoning shirts or zipping.
4. **Writing and Drawing:**
   - The development of fine motor skills is closely linked to learning to write and draw. The ability to draw clear and controlled lines, shape letters, and switch between pen or pencil grips are examples of fine motor skills.
5. **Manipulation of small parts:**
   - Fine motor skills are crucial for manipulating small objects. This may include opening screw caps, tying shoelaces, or assembling puzzles.
6. **Hand dexterity:**
   - Hand dexterity refers to the ability to perform complex actions that require coordinating different

hand movements. This includes activities such as cutting with scissors, folding paper, or doing crafts.
7. **Grafomotor skills:**
    - Grafomotor skills combine fine motor skills with visual perception skills and involve the coordination of hand and eye movements in written or drawing tasks.

Fine motor skills play a crucial role in child development and remain important for many everyday activities in adulthood. In occupational therapy, targeted interventions can be used to promote fine motor skills and support their development, especially in people with developmental disorders, neurological disorders, or injuries.

Forearm crutches

Forearm crutches, also known as elbow braces or forearm braces, are orthopedic aids designed to support the mobility of people with walking problems or temporary impairments. Unlike traditional walking sticks, which are primarily based on wrists and hands, forearm crutches support the user through a cuff that wraps around the forearm. Here are some key features and uses of forearm crutches:

1. **Cuff:** Instead of a handle, forearm crutches have a wide cuff that wraps around the user's forearm. This cuff provides more stability and support.
2. **Height adjustability:** As with traditional crutches, forearm crutches are usually height-adjustable to adapt to the user's individual height.
3. **Handle Design:** The grip area of the forearm crutches can be ergonomically designed to improve comfort and handling. Some models have a padded area for extra comfort.
4. **Non-slip rubber feet:** The ends of the forearm crutches are equipped with non-slip rubber feet to ensure stability while walking.
5. **Indications:** Forearm crutches are often used for injuries, surgeries, joint problems or other temporary walking impairments. They provide support when walking and help relieve body weight.
6. **Education:** It is important that individuals who use forearm crutches receive proper training and guidance to ensure that they can use the crutches correctly and effectively. This can help prevent falls or further injuries.

Forearm crutches are especially useful for people who need more stability than traditional walking sticks can provide. They allow for better weight distribution and can help reduce pressure on the wrists and hands.

Frustration tolerance

Frustration tolerance refers to a person's ability to deal constructively with frustration, discomfort, or disappointing events without causing excessive emotional distress or impulsive behavior. It is an important aspect of emotional intelligence and influences how people respond to challenges and stress.

Some characteristics of frustration tolerance include:

1. **Patience:** The ability to remain calm in difficult situations and wait for things to develop or improve.
2. **Acceptance of uncertainty:** The willingness to accept uncertainties and unpredictability without being overly unsettled.
3. **Flexibility:** The ability to adapt to changing circumstances and find alternative solutions when initial expectations are not met.
4. **Self-control:** The ability to avoid impulsive reactions and instead act thoughtfully and purposefully.
5. **Change of perspective:** The ability to look at a situation from different angles and understand other people's perspectives.
6. **Dealing with failure:** The ability to learn from failures rather than seeing them as personal defeats.

A high tolerance for frustration is important for managing stress, maintaining interpersonal relationships, and effectively dealing with professional or personal challenges. It also contributes to the development of endurance and resilience.

Frustration tolerance can be developed and strengthened through a variety of means, including:

1. **Mindfulness and self-reflection:** The conscious perception of feelings and the ability to understand one's own reaction to frustration.

2. **Relaxation techniques:** Techniques such as deep breathing, meditation, or progressive muscle relaxation can help reduce the emotional response to stress.
3. **Cognitive restructuring:** The ability to identify negative thought patterns and replace them with more positive or realistic ways of thinking.
4. **Problem-oriented coping strategies:** Actively addressing the root causes of frustration and seeking concrete solutions.
5. **Social support:** Sharing with other people can help broaden perspectives and provide emotional support.

The development of frustration tolerance is a continuous process that is influenced by personal experience, learning, and conscious effort.

Functional analysis

Functional analysis in occupational therapy refers to the systematic process of assessing and studying a person's individual abilities and limitations in relation to their daily activities and functions. The main objective of functional analysis is to develop a comprehensive understanding of the physical, cognitive, emotional and social aspects of a person in order to work specifically in the therapeutic intervention.

Functional analysis usually involves several steps:

1. **Anamnesis:** This involves gathering information about medical history, current state of health, life history, and individual life circumstances.
2. **Observation:** Through careful observation, the person's day-to-day activities and actions are analyzed. This can be done both in the clinical setting and in the real-life context.
3. **Assessment of activities and tasks.** The occupational therapist assesses the person's abilities in relation to specific activities of daily living (ADLs), instrumental activities of daily living (IADLs), or other specific tasks that are meaningful to the patient.
4. **Functional tests:** In some cases, standardized tests and assessment tools can be used to measure specific functional skills.
5. **Communication with the patient:** Throughout the process, communication with the patient is crucial. Understanding the individual's personal goals, needs, and ideas is key.

The results of the functional analysis serve as the basis for the formulation of an individual treatment plan in occupational therapy. This plan aims to improve the autonomy, independence and quality of life of the individual through targeted interventions.

Functional training

Functional training refers to specific exercises and interventions aimed at improving the functions of the body, especially after injuries, illnesses or surgical procedures. It is widely used in rehabilitation to promote mobility, strength, endurance, and other functional skills. Functional training can be applied in various areas of health care, including physical therapy and occupational therapy. The functional training consists of:

1. **Targeted exercises:**
   - Functional training includes targeted exercises aimed at improving specific functions of the body. This can include strengthening certain muscles, improving joint mobility, or promoting coordinated movements.
2. **Individualization:**
   - The exercises in functional training are often individually adapted to the needs and abilities of the individual. Therapy goals are determined based on the patient's specific diagnosis and personal goals.
3. **Rehabilitation after injuries or surgeries:**
   - Functional training is often used to support rehabilitation after injuries, orthopedic procedures, or other surgical procedures. This may include restoring mobility, strength, and function to the affected area.
4. **Coordination and balance:**
   - An important part of functional training is the improvement of coordination and balance. This is particularly relevant for patients after neurological events such as stroke or in the elderly who have an increased risk of falling.
5. **Endurance training:**
   - Functional training can also include endurance exercises to promote cardiovascular fitness and overall endurance. This is important for coping with daily activities and participating in social life.

6. **Everyday activities:**
    - In some cases, everyday activities are integrated into functional training. This could be lifting objects, climbing stairs, or other movements relevant to daily life.
7. **Progressive loading:**
    - Functional training often involves a progressive increase in load to ensure the steady improvement of functions. This may include the gradual increase in resistance, the intensity of exercises, or the duration of activities.
8. **Patient involvement:**
    - An important aspect of functional training is the patient's involvement in their own healing process. The understanding of the exercises and the active participation of the patient are crucial for the success of functional training.

Functional training is used by various professionals such as physical therapists and occupational therapists and plays a crucial role in restoring functionality after health challenges.

Gait analysis

Gait analysis is a specific area of occupational therapy that focuses on examining and evaluating a person's gait pattern. Understanding gait analysis is important to identify limitations, difficulties, or potential problems related to locomotion. This process plays a crucial role in the development of interventions to improve the mobility and independence of the individual. Here are some characteristics that are considered in a gait analysis:

1. **Stride cycle:** Gait analysis looks at the different phases of the stride cycle, including foot touchdown, roll, foot pulling, and bounce phase. The analysis of these phases helps to identify possible deviations or abnormalities.
2. **Posture and alignment:** The person's posture while walking is observed to see if there are any deviations or irregularities. This includes the alignment of the head, shoulders, spine, hips, and legs.
3. **Foot attachment pattern:** The way the foot is placed on the floor is analyzed. This can help identify problems such as supinated or pronated foot strike, toe or heel running.
4. **Stride size and stride length:** The size and length of the steps are measured and analyzed. Abnormalities may indicate muscle weakness, balance problems, or other factors.
5. **Speed:** The speed of walking is evaluated to determine if the person is able to maintain an appropriate pace and if assistance may be required.
6. **Balance and coordination:** Gait analysis can also assess balance and coordination while walking. This is important to minimize the risk of falling and ensure the safety of the person.

The information from gait analysis allows occupational therapists to plan targeted interventions to improve their patients' mobility, stability, and independence. This may include exercises to strengthen muscles, balance exercises, adjustments to walking aids, or other therapeutic measures.

Geriatrics

Geriatrics is the medical specialty that deals with the prevention, diagnosis, treatment, and rehabilitation of diseases and dysfunction in the elderly. It is designed to promote health, independence and quality of life in old age. Geriatrics is interdisciplinary and often involves various health professions, including doctors, nurses, physical therapists, occupational therapists, and social workers.

Features of geriatrics include:

1. **Multimorbidity:** Older people tend to be more likely to suffer from multiple health problems occurring at the same time. Geriatrics takes this multimorbidity into account and develops holistic treatment approaches.
2. **Functional preservation:** A central goal of geriatrics is to maintain or improve the functional abilities of older people. These include mobility, cognitive function, sensory abilities, and the ability to take care of themselves.
3. **Prevention of the need for long-term care:** Geriatrics is actively committed to avoiding the need for long-term care. This can be achieved through early detection and interventions for health problems, as well as by promoting a healthy lifestyle.
4. **Medication management:** Due to aging processes, older people may be more susceptible to drug interactions and side effects. Geriatrics deals with adapted medication management to ensure that older people receive the right medications at appropriate dosages.
5. **Geriatric teams:** Caring for the elderly often requires the collaboration of different professionals. Geriatric teams, which may consist of doctors, nurses, therapists, and social workers, work together to provide comprehensive care.
6. **Age-associated diseases:** Geriatrics is specifically concerned with age-associated diseases such as dementia, osteoporosis, cardiovascular disease, and other health problems that are more common in older age.

In geriatrics, the focus is on the individual consideration of the elderly. The therapeutic approaches are designed to improve quality of life, promote independence and ensure the best possible health in old age.

Gerontology

Gerontology is a scientific discipline that deals with the process of aging and its related aspects on a physical, psychological and social level. Unlike geriatrics, which focuses on the medical care of the elderly, gerontology views aging as a multidimensional phenomenon and explores it from different perspectives.

Aspects of gerontology are:

1. **Biological dimension:** Gerontology studies biological aspects of aging, including changes in cells, tissues, and organs. She also researches genetic factors that can influence aging.
2. **Psychological dimension:** Psychological gerontology deals with the emotional, cognitive, and psychosocial changes that can occur with age. The focus is on topics such as memory, emotional health, personality development and life satisfaction.
3. **Sociological dimension:** Sociological gerontology looks at the impact of ageing on social structures, social relationships, and the role of older people in society. She explores social challenges and opportunities related to aging.
4. **Epidemiology of Aging:** Gerontology studies demographic patterns, health trends, and the prevalence of disease in the elderly. This helps to better understand the needs of the ageing population.
5. **Geron technology:** An emerging field in gerontology is geron technology, which deals with the development and application of technologies to improve the quality of life of the elderly and promote their independence.
6. **Long-term care and care systems:** Gerontology also explores the structures and challenges associated with long-term care and care systems, including the development of services and support systems for the elderly.

Gerontology is interdisciplinary, drawing on findings from various disciplines such as medicine, psychology, sociology, biology, and others. Its aim is to deepen the understanding of ageing in order to improve the quality of life of older people and to better adapt health and social policies to their needs.

Group therapy

Group therapy is a form of psychotherapy in which a small group of people work together on their emotional, social, or psychological challenges. Under the guidance of a qualified therapist, group therapy provides a safe space where members can share their experiences, receive support, and work together on personal growth and change. Some features of group therapy:

1. **Group dynamics:** Group dynamics play a crucial role in group therapy. The interactions between the members, their relationships with each other, and the way they interact with each other influence the therapeutic process.
2. **Universality:** Group therapy emphasizes the idea of universality, which means that many individual problems and experiences can be shared by others in the group. This can help reduce feelings of isolation and foster an understanding of common human challenges.
3. **Sharing experiences:** Participating in a group allows members to share their own stories, emotions, and perspectives. By listening to others, they can learn about different points of view and coping strategies.
4. **Group process:** The group process refers to the way the group interacts with each other, develops, and deals with the challenges. Therapists observe and guide this process to further therapeutic goals.
5. **Support and feedback:** Groups provide a supportive community where members can encourage each other. At the same time, the group also facilitates constructive feedback that can contribute to self-reflection and change.
6. **Diversity of perspectives:** In a group, people with different backgrounds, life experiences and personalities come together. This diversity can offer a wide range of perspectives and solutions to individual problems.
7. **Efficiency and cost:** Group therapy can be more efficient and reduce costs compared to individual therapy because several people are supported at the same time. This is especially important when resources are limited.

8. **Confidentiality:** Group therapy is based on a principle of confidentiality, similar to individual therapy. Members are committed to respecting each other's privacy and stories.

Group therapy can be effective for a variety of problems, including depression, anxiety disorders, relationship problems, addiction, trauma, and other mental health issues. The dynamics and benefits may vary depending on the group composition and therapeutic approach.

Group work

Group work refers to people working together in a group to achieve common goals, accomplish tasks, or solve problems. Group work can occur in a variety of contexts, be it school projects, professional settings, non-profit organizations, or other social settings. Aspects of group work:

1. **Collaboration and interaction:** Group work emphasizes collaboration and interaction between members. It's about people sharing their skills, knowledge, and perspectives to work effectively together.
2. **Goals and tasks:** Groups usually have specific goals or tasks that they need to achieve. These can range from solving a problem, to creating a product, to implementing projects.
3. **Distribution of roles:** Different roles can arise in group work to promote efficiency and productivity. These include, for example, the organizer, the idea provider, the coordinator or the time manager.
4. **Communication: Communication** is a key element in group work. Effective communication allows for the exchange of information, the clarification of tasks and the resolution of conflicts.
5. **Conflict management:** Conflicts can occur in group work, whether due to differing opinions, unclear communication, or other factors. Effective conflict management is important to ensure a smooth workflow.
6. **Motivation and commitment:** The motivation of the group members plays a crucial role in the success of the group work. A positive working atmosphere and the recognition of individual contributions contribute to motivation.
7. **Learning processes:** In school or professional contexts, group work also serves as a learning tool. Members can learn from each other, improve their skills, and gain new perspectives.
8. **Results-oriented:** Group work aims to achieve concrete results. These could be presentations, reports, products, or other results generated by the group's collective efforts.

Group work can provide many benefits, including improved creativity, the use of different skills and perspectives, and the promotion of social skills. However, it also requires a clear structure, communication, and effective collaboration to be successful.

Hand Therapy

Hand therapy is a specialized field of physical therapy or occupational therapy that focuses on the rehabilitation of people with injuries, illnesses, or dysfunctions in the hands, wrists, arms, and sometimes shoulders. The aim of hand therapy is to improve the function and dexterity of the hands, reduce pain and restore patients' independence in their daily lives. Information on hand therapy:

1. **Evaluation and diagnosis:** Hand therapists perform a comprehensive evaluation to identify the exact cause of the hand problems. This can include injuries such as fractures, tendon injuries, arthritis, or neurological disorders.
2. **Individual therapy plan:** Based on the diagnosis, the hand therapist creates an individual therapy plan. This plan may include exercises, manual therapy, ergonomic adjustments, splints, and other interventions.
3. **Pain management:** Pain reduction is often an important part of hand therapy. This can be achieved through targeted exercises, manual techniques, modalities such as heat or cold, and splints or bandages.
4. **Improve mobility and strength:** Hand therapists work to improve joint mobility and strength in the hands. This can be achieved through targeted exercises and progressive exercise programs.
5. **Scar management:** Injuries, surgeries, or burns can cause scarring, which can affect the mobility and function of the hands. Hand therapy may include methods of scar massage and stretching to improve tissue flexibility.
6. **Fine motor skills training:** Hand therapy often focuses on improving fine motor skills that are important for everyday tasks such as writing, typing, grasping small objects, and other actions.
7. **Adaptation and ergonomics:** Hand therapists can make recommendations for ergonomic adjustments in the workplace or at home to minimize repetitive strain and promote healing.

8. **Patient education:** An important aspect of hand therapy is patient education. Patients learn how to protect their hands, perform exercises at home, and maintain their hand health in the long term.

Hand therapy is often performed by physical therapists or occupational therapists who specialize in this specialty. They often work closely with surgeons, rheumatologists, and other health care providers to provide comprehensive care for people with hand problems.

Handcrafts

Hand skills refer to the skills and dexterity that a person possesses in the use of the hands and fingers. These skills are important for a variety of daily activities and can range from coarse motor movements to fine motor tasks. Here are some aspects and examples of manual skills:

1. **Fine motor skills:** Fine motor skills refer to the precise control of small muscles, especially in the hands and fingers. This includes activities such as grasping small objects, writing, closing buttons, or operating a computer mouse.
2. **Gross motor skills:** Gross motor skills refer to the coordination and control of larger muscle groups that are responsible for gross movements. This includes activities such as walking, running, jumping, throwing, or lifting heavy objects.
3. **Dexterity in craftsmanship and art:** Creative activities often require strong hand skills. Examples include painting, drawing, carving, sewing, knitting, and other handicraft activities that require precise hand movements.
4. **Instrument playing:** Playing musical instruments requires a high level of manual dexterity, whether it's fingering strings on a guitar, beating drums, or playing keyboard instruments.
5. **Sporting activities:** Many sports activities require strong manual skills. For example, in tennis, holding and hitting the ball, in basketball, dribbling and passing, or in climbing, grabbing rocks.
6. **Everyday activities:** Simple daily activities often require manual skills, such as opening a bottle, cutting food with a knife, tying shoelaces, or operating household appliances.
7. **Hand skills in children:** The development of hand skills in children is an important part of their early education. Activities such as playing with building blocks, painting, putting puzzles together, and crafting promote the development of fine motor skills.

The development of hand skills often occurs throughout life through learning, practicing, and participating in various activities. Fostering these skills is important to support independence, self-sufficiency, and participation in different areas of life.

Hand-eye coordination

Hand-eye coordination refers to the body's ability to perceive visual information and then perform precise and coordinated movements of the hands. It is an essential aspect for a variety of everyday activities and plays an important role in various fields, including sports, crafts, professional activities, and many others.

Here are some key points about hand-eye coordination:

1. **Visual perception:** The ability to capture and interpret visual stimuli is crucial for hand-eye coordination. This includes processing information about distances, speeds, sizes, and shapes.
2. **Precise movements:** Hand-eye coordination enables precise and purposeful hand movements. This is especially important for tasks that require accurate handling of tools, instruments, or other objects.
3. **Fine motor skills:** The ability to precisely control small muscles, especially in the hands and fingers, is called fine motor skills and is closely related to hand-eye coordination. Fine motor skills are necessary for activities such as writing, drawing, sewing, or operating small switches and buttons.
4. **Gross motor skills:** Although hand-eye coordination is often associated with fine motor skills, it also plays a role in gross motor movements. This includes activities such as catching a ball, throwing objects, or walking along a narrow path.
5. **Developmental stages:** Hand-eye coordination develops at different stages in the course of a child's development. Early childhood activities such as grasping objects, coordinating eye movements, and exploring objects contribute to the development of this skill.
6. **Training and improvement:** Hand-eye coordination can be improved through targeted training. This may include exercises, games, or activities specifically aimed at strengthening the connection between visual perception and hand movements.

7. **Professional importance:** In many professional fields, such as surgery, crafts, sports or computer work, effective hand-eye coordination is of great importance. It can affect work performance, efficiency, and safety.

Hand-eye coordination plays an important role not only in professional contexts, but also in daily life. It helps us to successfully cope with tasks that require precise collaboration of visual and motor skills.

Hemiparesis

Hemiparesis refers to partial paralysis that affects only one side of the body. The term "hemi" means "half," and "paresis" stands for impaired muscle function or muscle weakness. Hemiparesis often occurs as a result of damage to the central nervous system, especially the brain.

The most common cause of hemiparesis is stroke. When a person suffers a stroke, it can lead to impaired blood flow in the brain, which in turn leads to damage to nerve cells. Depending on which region of the brain is affected, this can lead to hemiparesis.

Symptoms of hemiparesis may include:

1. **Muscle weakness:** The affected side of the body may be weak or paralyzed.
2. **Impaired fine motor skills:** difficulty with precise movements, such as grasping or writing.
3. **Balance problems:** The ability to maintain balance and walk may be impaired.
4. **Changes in muscle tension:** Increased or decreased muscle tension may occur.
5. **Limited range of motion:** The mobility of the affected limbs may be restricted.

Rehabilitation of hemiparesis focuses on supporting the affected person in their functionality, improving mobility and promoting their independence in everyday life. This can be achieved through physical therapy, occupational therapy, and speech therapy, depending on the specific needs of the person. The prognosis depends on several factors, including the cause of the hemiparesis, the extent of the damage, and the underlying health of the affected person. However, early intervention and comprehensive rehabilitation treatment can help improve functioning and optimize quality of life.

Hemiplegia

Hemiplegia is a medical term that refers to the complete paralysis of one side of the body, usually on one side of the body. This condition often occurs as a result of damage to the central nervous system, especially the brain or spinal cord. The impairment can be triggered by various causes such as stroke, traumatic brain injury, tumors or neurological diseases.

Hemiplegia usually affects the arms, legs, and often the face on one side of the body. The severity of paralysis can vary, from mild limitations to complete immobility. People with hemiplegia may have difficulty walking, grasping, holding objects, or other everyday activities.

In occupational therapy, the rehabilitation of patients with hemiplegia plays a crucial role. The therapeutic goals include the restoration of motor skills, the promotion of independence in daily activities and the adaptation to the changed life circumstances. Occupational therapists use various methods, exercises, and techniques to improve the functioning of the affected side of the body and help patients improve their quality of life.

Holistic Approach

A holistic approach, also known as a holistic approach, refers to looking at a system as a whole, where the pieces are connected to each other and work together to understand the entire system. This approach assumes that the whole is greater than the sum of its parts and that understanding and intervention at all levels are necessary to promote the well-being and functioning of the system. The holistic approach is applied in various fields, including medicine, psychology, nutrition, education, and environmental sciences. Here are some basic characteristics of the holistic approach:

1. **Holistic understanding:** A holistic approach strives to develop a comprehensive understanding of a system by not only looking at the individual parts in isolation, but also by considering the interactions between the parts and their impact on the overall system.
2. **Body, mind and soul:** In medicine and health care, the holistic approach often refers to the consideration of body, mind and spirit as an inseparable unit. This means that physical health, mental well-being, and emotional balance are considered together to understand an individual's health.
3. **Individual in context:** In psychology and psychotherapy, the holistic approach is applied to understanding the individual in the context of his or her social, cultural and environmental factors. This allows for a more comprehensive diagnosis and intervention.
4. **Environment and sustainability:** In the field of environmental science, a holistic approach can mean looking not only at the individual environmental components, but also at their interactions and impacts on the ecosystem and society.
5. **Holistic nutrition:** In nutrition, a holistic approach refers to emphasizing a balanced diet that takes into account not only nutrients but also other factors such as eating habits, lifestyle, and environmental conditions.
6. **Pedagogy:** In education, a holistic approach can mean looking at students as a whole, including their cognitive,

social, emotional, and physical development. The curriculum may aim to promote different aspects of the personality.
7. **Spirituality:** For some people, a holistic approach can also include spiritual dimensions, integrating the search for meaning and purpose in life into the holistic view.
8. **Preventative approaches:** Holistic approaches often emphasize preventative measures and lifestyle factors to promote well-being and prevent disease, rather than just focusing on treating symptoms.

The holistic approach is therefore a way of looking at things that aims to grasp the complexity and multi-layered nature of systems, whether in the human body, in social communities, in the environment or in other contexts.

Hydrotherapy

Hydrotherapy is a form of therapy that uses water in various forms and temperatures as a therapeutic medium. This form of therapy is used in various medical, rehabilitative and wellness-oriented contexts. Features of hydrotherapy:

1. **Water Applications:** Hydrotherapy includes a variety of water treatments, including baths, showers, Kneipp treatments, wraps, compresses, and other techniques.
2. **Temperature variations:** A characteristic feature of hydrotherapy is the variation of water temperatures. Warm, cold and cold-blooded applications can have different therapeutic effects.
3. **Relaxation and stress relief:** Warm water treatments can help relax muscles, reduce stress, and promote overall relaxation. Warm baths, for example, are a common form of hydrotherapy.
4. **Promoting blood circulation:** Warm water applications can promote blood circulation, which can have positive effects on metabolism and oxygenation of tissues.
5. **Muscle pain relief:** Hydrotherapy can help relieve muscle pain, tension, and stiffness, especially after injuries or strenuous physical activity.
6. **Rehabilitation:** In rehabilitation after injuries or surgeries, hydrotherapy can be used to improve mobility, strengthen muscles, and aid in the healing process.
7. **Cold water applications:** Cold water applications can be used to reduce inflammation, swelling and promote wound healing.
8. **Kneipp treatments:** The Kneipp treatments developed by Sebastian Kneipp are a special form of hydrotherapy that involves alternating between cold and warm water. These treatments are said to boost the immune system and promote overall health.
9. **Aquatherapy:** In aquatherapy, special exercises are performed in water to improve physical functions, strengthen muscles and promote flexibility.

10. **Wellness treatments:** Apart from medical and rehabilitative purposes, hydrotherapy is often used in the wellness sector as well. Hot tubs, thermal baths, and spa treatments can help relax and rejuvenate.

It should be noted that hydrotherapy can vary depending on a person's individual needs and condition. The use of this form of therapy should ideally be done under the guidance of professionals such as physiotherapists, doctors or spa therapists to ensure that it meets the specific requirements.

Hypertension

Hypertension is a medical term used to describe permanently elevated blood pressure. Blood pressure is the pressure of circulating blood on the walls of blood vessels. It is expressed by two values: systolic pressure (the higher value during cardiac contraction) and diastolic pressure (the lower value during cardiac relaxation).

Usually, blood pressure is measured in millimeters of mercury (mmHg). Normal blood pressure is usually around 120/80 mmHg. Hypertension is when blood pressure is persistently above what is considered normal. A distinction is made between different degrees:

1. **Mild hypertension (stage 1):** blood pressure between 140-159/90-99 mmHg
2. **Moderate hypertension (stage 2):** blood pressure between 160-179/100-109 mmHg
3. **Severe hypertension (stage 3):** blood pressure from 180/110 mmHg

Hypertension is a significant risk factor for various cardiovascular diseases, including stroke, heart attack, heart failure, and kidney failure. However, there are often no obvious symptoms, which is why hypertension is called the "silent killer". Therefore, it is important to monitor blood pressure regularly to detect and treat hypertension early. Treatment for hypertension can include various approaches, including lifestyle changes such as a healthy diet, regular physical activity, smoking cessation, and weight management. In some cases, drug therapy may also be necessary. The exact treatment strategy is tailored to the individual patient, depending on factors such as the degree of hypertension, comorbidities and other individual health aspects. It is important to take hypertension seriously and seek medical attention to avoid possible complications.

Hypotension

Hypotension is the medical term for low blood pressure. Similar to hypertension, the high blood pressure, hypotension is a condition that concerns the pressure of circulating blood on the walls of blood vessels.

Normal blood pressure is typically around 120/80 mmHg. Hypotension occurs when blood pressure drops permanently below these normal values. However, there are no clear categories for mild, moderate or severe hypotension as in hypertension. Low blood pressure alone is usually not as problematic as high blood pressure unless it causes symptoms.

Symptoms of hypotension can include dizziness, lightheadedness, fainting, difficulty concentrating, fatigue and, in some cases, blurred vision. There are various causes of hypotension, including dehydration, heart problems, hormonal changes, side effects of medications, or simply genetic predisposition.

Treatment of hypotension depends on the cause. In many cases, lifestyle changes can help, such as adequate fluid intake, regular physical activity, adjusting eating habits, and avoiding excessive alcohol consumption. In some cases, it may be necessary to treat the underlying cause of hypotension, for example by treating heart problems or adjusting medications.

Inclusion

Inclusion refers to the principle that all people, regardless of their individual characteristics, backgrounds, or abilities, have the right to participate fully in all areas of society. This term is in contrast to exclusion and discriminatory practices. Inclusion strives to create a society in which diversity is accepted, valued and seen as an enrichment. Here are some key concepts related to inclusion:

1. **Diversity:** Inclusion recognizes and values the diversity of human characteristics, backgrounds, and abilities, including but not limited to gender, age, ethnicity, religion, sexual orientation, physical and mental abilities.
2. **Equal opportunities:** Inclusion strives for equal opportunities for all. This means that every person should have equal opportunities to participate in education, work, social activities, and other areas of life.
3. **Accessibility:** Inclusion also means removing barriers that miqht prevent people from living a full life in society. These include physical barriers, communicative barriers, stereotypes, and other forms of discrimination.
4. **Participation:** Inclusion goes beyond mere presence and involves the active participation of all people in the various aspects of society, whether in schools, workplaces, communities or cultural events.
5. **A sense of community:** Inclusion fosters a sense of community where each person is respected and feels an integral part of the community. It emphasizes the importance of social integration and cooperation.
6. **Education:** In inclusive education, this means that all children, regardless of their abilities or differences, should be taught together in regular schools. Individual needs and support are taken into account.
7. **Workplace:** Inclusion in the workplace involves creating environments that are accessible to people with different abilities and providing appropriate adaptations to ensure that all employees can succeed.

8. **Societal change:** Inclusion often requires social change based on prejudices, stereotypes, and discriminatory structures. The goal is to create a society that values and promotes diversity.

Inclusion is a comprehensive approach that requires not only individual change, but also societal and institutional adjustments. It is a positive vision that aims to create a society in which every person experiences equal rights, opportunities and recognition.

Increased effectiveness

Increasing effectiveness in the context of occupational therapy refers to improving the effectiveness and efficiency of therapeutic interventions in order to achieve optimal outcomes for patients. In occupational therapy, increasing effectiveness can be achieved in several ways:

1. **Individualization of therapy:** Each patient has different needs, abilities and goals. By adapting the therapy to the individual circumstances of the patient, the effectiveness can be increased.
2. **Use of evidence-based practices:** The use of methods and interventions based on scientific evidence and research will help ensure that therapy is effective. This means that the approaches used can demonstrably achieve positive results.
3. **Ongoing evaluation and adjustment:** Regular review of the patient's progress allows the occupational therapist to adjust therapy plans as needed. This flexible customization is critical to ensure that interventions meet the patient's current needs.
4. **Promoting self-reliance:** Occupational therapy often aims to promote patient autonomy and independence. Increasing effectiveness can be achieved by the therapy aimed at strengthening patients' skills and resources to be able to carry out their daily activities independently.
5. **Interdisciplinary collaboration:** Effective collaboration with other healthcare providers, such as doctors, nurses, and other therapists, can improve the overall effectiveness of treatment. A holistic approach supports patients in various aspects of their health.

The increase in effectiveness in occupational therapy is thus aimed at optimizing the quality of therapy in order to achieve the best possible results for patients.

Individual Therapy

Individual therapy, also known as one-on-one therapy or one-on-one talk therapy, refers to a form of psychotherapeutic treatment in which an individual works with a therapist in a confidential setting. This form of therapy allows individuals to explore and manage personal concerns, challenges, or mental health issues. Here are some key features of individual therapy:

1. **Confidentiality:** Individual therapy provides a safe space where privacy and confidentiality are maintained. This allows individuals to talk openly about personal experiences and emotions.
2. **Individualized:** The therapy is tailored to the individual needs, goals and challenges of the client. The therapist tailors the interventions to address the specific concerns of the individual.
3. **Therapeutic alliance:** An important part of individual therapy is the establishment of a therapeutic alliance between the client and the therapist. The relationship between the two is crucial to the success of the therapy.
4. **Diagnosis and treatment plan:** The therapist can make a diagnostic assessment if necessary and develop an individualized treatment plan. This plan may include different therapeutic approaches and techniques, depending on the goals of the therapy.
5. **Self-exploration:** Individual therapy offers space for self-exploration and self-reflection. The client has the opportunity to understand their thoughts, feelings and behavioral patterns and to bring about positive changes.
6. **Coping strategies:** The therapist can help the client develop effective coping strategies to deal with life challenges, stress, anxiety, or other mental health issues.
7. **Emotional support:** Individual therapy provides a supportive environment in which the client can express their emotions. The therapist can help process negative emotions and promote positive emotions.

8. **Long-term or short-term therapy:** The duration of individual therapy may vary. Some therapies are short-term and aim to address specific concerns, while other therapies are long-term and promote deeper personal development.
9. **Psychoeducation:** The therapist can provide information and psychoeducational elements to allow the client to have a better understanding of their own mental health, relationships, or other relevant issues.
10. **Nurturing resources:** Individual therapy can aim to nurture and leverage the client's individual resources, strengths, and abilities to support positive change.

There are various therapeutic approaches in individual therapy, including cognitive-behavioral therapy, psychodynamic therapy, humanistic therapy, and many others. The choice of approach depends on the needs of the client and the goals of the therapy.

Instrumental Activities of Daily Living (IADL)

Instrumental activities of daily living (IADL) refer to complex, more demanding everyday activities that are important for self-reliance and self-determined living in the community. Unlike the so-called activities of daily living (ADL), which involve basic self-care tasks, IADLs are more complex and often require higher cognitive skills. These concepts are often used in the context of health and social care and occupational therapy. Here are some examples of instrumental activities of daily living:

1. **Shopping:** This includes not only shopping for groceries, but also the ability to compare prices, create shopping lists, manage budgets, and organize the transportation of purchases.
2. **Cooking and preparing meals:** This is not only about preparing food, but also about understanding recipes, planning meals, knowing nutritional principles, and how to use kitchen appliances safely.
3. **Housework:** This includes tasks such as cleaning, vacuuming, doing laundry, making beds, and general housekeeping. Planning skills, organizational skills and physical resilience are important here.
4. **Financial management:** The ability to manage financial matters, pay bills, prepare budgets, conduct banking, and other financial responsibilities also falls within the purview of IADL.
5. **Transportation:** This includes planning and organizing travel, using public transport, driving a vehicle, and ensuring mobility in the community.
6. **Communication:** Using phones, computers, and other means of communication, composing emails, reading newspapers, and understanding written information are important IADLs.
7. **Medication management:** Proper medication intake, knowledge of dosages, and adherence to medical instructions are key elements of IADL in the health context.
8. **Self-care and personal hygiene:** Although basic personal hygiene is part of the activities of daily living, more complex

aspects such as styling hair, nail care, and choosing clothes can also be part of the IADL.

IADLs play an important role in assessing the functional abilities of the elderly or those with health restrictions. Support at IADL is a goal of rehabilitation and care in order to maintain or improve the independence and quality of life of those affected. Occupational therapists often specialize in helping people develop or restore these skills.

Interdisciplinary collaboration

Interdisciplinary collaboration refers to the cooperation and exchange of experts from different disciplines or professional fields in order to work together on complex problems or challenges. In many fields, especially healthcare, education, research and social services, interdisciplinary collaboration has become increasingly important as it helps to develop more comprehensive and holistic solutions. Here are some key features of interdisciplinary collaboration:

1. **Different disciplines:** Interdisciplinary collaboration involves professionals from different disciplines or disciplines to bring different perspectives, methods, and expertise to the solution approach. These can be, for example, health scientists, psychologists, social workers, educators or technicians.
2. **Shared goals:** All professionals involved work together on an overarching goal or problem. This could include improving patient care in healthcare, developing innovative solutions in technology, or promoting student education and development in the school sector.
3. **Communication and exchange:** Effective communication is crucial for interdisciplinary collaboration. Professionals need to communicate openly with each other to share their perspectives, share information, and work collaboratively on solutions.
4. **Holistic approach:** Interdisciplinary collaboration enables a holistic approach to solving complex problems. By integrating different expertise, more comprehensive and coordinated solutions can be developed.
5. **Respect for diversity:** Since different disciplines have different perspectives and approaches, interdisciplinary collaboration requires respect for diversity and recognition of the different contributions of each team member.
6. **Increased efficiency:** The collaboration of professionals from different fields can lead to a more efficient use of resources. By sharing expertise, problems can be solved faster and more effectively.

7. **Development of new ideas:** The diversity of expertise and perspectives in an interdisciplinary team can foster creativity and enable the development of new ideas or approaches.
8. **Considering complexity:** Many modern problems are complex and require deep understanding from different angles. Interdisciplinary collaboration makes it possible to better understand and address the complexity of problems.

Examples of interdisciplinary collaboration can be found in various contexts, including healthcare teams, research projects, educational initiatives, and innovation projects in business. Successful interdisciplinary collaboration requires openness, teamwork and the ability to think across disciplinary boundaries.

International Classification of Functioning, Disability and Health (ICF)

The International Classification of Functioning, Disability and Health (ICF) is a classification system developed by the World Health Organization (WHO). It serves to expand and improve the understanding of health and related conditions. The ICF was first published in 2001 and is an internationally accepted standard that is used worldwide in healthcare, research and policy.

The ICF consists of two main parts:

1. **Functionality and disability:**
   - **Body functions and structures:** This area includes anatomical structures of the body (e.g., organs, limbs) and physiological functions (e.g., vision, hearing, movement functions).
   - **Activities and participation:** This describes the activities that a person performs (e.g. walking, reading) and their participation in social areas (e.g. work, education, social activities).
2. **Contextual factors:**
   - **Environmental factors:** This area looks at external factors that can affect a person's life, including physical environment (e.g., architecture, climate), personal support (e.g., family, social environment), and political and social systems.
   - **Personal factors:** These include individual characteristics such as gender, age, lifestyle, habits and social backgrounds.

The ICF uses a bio-psycho-social approach that emphasizes the interactions between biological, psychological, and social factors in determining health and functioning. It is not limited to the description of diseases or impairments, but considers the state of health as a complex interplay of various influencing factors.

The ICF is applied in various areas:

- **Healthcare:** To classify diagnoses, plan rehabilitation interventions, and evaluate the effectiveness of interventions.
- **Research:** To enable a standardized and comparable description of health conditions in different studies.
- **Social policy:** To develop strategies to promote the participation of people with disabilities and to create accessible environments.

The ICF has helped promote a more comprehensive and inclusive approach to health care that goes beyond the traditional disease perspective and takes into account the importance of social and environmental aspects in assessing health and functioning.

Introspection

Self-awareness refers to a person's awareness and cognition of themselves, including their own feelings, thoughts, behaviors, strengths and weaknesses. It is a central aspect of emotional intelligence and a fundamental element for personal growth and self-development. More information about self-awareness:

1. **Self-reflection:**
    - Self-awareness includes the ability to self-reflect. This means that a person is able to think about their own thoughts, emotions, and actions.
2. **Awareness of one's own emotions:**
    - Self-awareness refers to the awareness of one's own emotions. This includes identifying, understanding, and accepting feelings.
3. **Self-knowledge:**
    - Self-awareness includes a deep understanding of one's personality, values, beliefs, goals, and motivations. It's about knowing who you are.
4. **Self-concept:**
    - The self-image or self-concept is an essential part of self-perception. It refers to how a person sees himself, what qualities he considers important, and how he defines his own identity.
5. **Acceptance of weaknesses:**
    - A healthy self-awareness includes the ability to recognize and accept weaknesses and mistakes without devaluing oneself.
6. **Self-criticism:**
    - Self-awareness also includes self-criticism, but in a constructive way. It means objectively assessing yourself and identifying opportunities for improvement without overly punishing yourself.
7. **Body Awareness:**
    - This refers to awareness of one's own body, needs and physical well-being. Positive body perception contributes to self-acceptance.

8. **Self-confidence:**
    - Self-awareness is closely related to self-confidence. A realistic understanding of one's own abilities and potential promotes healthy self-confidence.
9. **Self-determination:**
    - The ability for self-determination and self-leadership is another aspect of self-awareness. This means making conscious decisions and taking responsibility for one's own path in life.
10. **Readiness for development:**
    - A positive self-perception often goes hand in hand with a willingness to develop and change personally. It means being open to new experiences and learning opportunities.

A strong awareness of oneself forms the basis for effective interpersonal relationships, professional success, and personal well-being. Self-awareness is an ongoing process that is fostered by mindfulness, self-reflection, and a willingness to develop personally.

KAWA Model

The KAWA model is a concept in occupational therapy that was originally developed by Dr. Michael Iwama. "KAWA" is the Japanese word for "flow", and the model metaphorically deals with the flow of life, especially in terms of individual adaptation to change and challenges. The KAWA model is particularly useful in the cultural contextualization of occupational therapy and consideration of personal perspectives.

Here are some key concepts of the KAWA model:

1. **The River:** The river represents life and symbolizes the course of an individual's journey through life. It stands for the flow of life, constant change and adaptability.
2. **The River Environment:** This refers to the environment in which the river moves. It is the external conditions and contexts of life, including cultural, social, political and economic factors.
3. **The Stone Pathway:** This path runs alongside the river and represents a person's individual abilities, resources, and coping mechanisms. These stones affect the flow and can change over time.
4. **Personal Perspective:** This refers to the individual's perception of the river and its surroundings. Each person has their own unique view of their life and experiences.

The KAWA model is often used to integrate culture into therapeutic practice. It emphasizes the importance that individual perspective and cultural contexts have in designing interventions and supporting people in their life journey. Occupational therapists using the KAWA model are encouraged to respect the uniqueness of each individual, to consider cultural differences, and to work with the client to find ways to overcome challenges and promote individual well-being.

Kinaesthetics

Kinaesthetics is a concept that deals with the perception and design of movements. It was developed by the Swiss nursing scientist Dr. Frank Hatch and is mainly used in healthcare, especially in nursing, rehabilitation and in the field of health promotion. The term "kinaesthetics" is composed of the Greek words "kinesis" (movement) and "aisthesis" (perception) and thus emphasizes the connection between movement and perception.

Here are some basic concepts and principles of Kinaesthetics:

1. **Self-care literacy:** Kinaesthetics aims to promote people's self-care literacy. This includes the ability to perceive, control and optimize one's own movements.
2. **Movement as a Principle of Life:** The concept considers movement as a fundamental principle of life. By promoting conscious exercise, the quality of life and well-being are to be improved.
3. **Design of movements:** Kinaesthetics involves the targeted design of movements in order to enable an efficient and gentle execution of everyday activities. This can be relevant both for caring for patients and for supporting people in everyday life.
4. **Sensorimotor integration:** The concept emphasizes the integration of sensory (perceptual) and motor (movement) skills. By training this integration, people can improve and optimize their movements.
5. **Motion perception:** Kinaesthetics attaches great importance to the perception of movement. This includes the conscious experience of how movements begin, progress and end, as well as attention to one's own posture.
6. **Avoidance of overload:** One goal of Kinaesthetics is to avoid overloads and incorrect loads. This is achieved by training efficient movement sequences in order to minimize the strain on the musculoskeletal system.
7. **Individuality:** Kinaesthetics takes into account the individuality of each person. The movement sequences and

strategies are individually adapted to the needs, abilities and goals.
8. **Use in various fields:** Kinaesthetics is used not only in healthcare, but also in other fields such as education, occupational therapy, and rehabilitation.
9. **Training of professionals:** Healthcare professionals, especially nurses, are trained in kinaesthetics to be able to apply the principles in their daily work.

Kinaesthetics thus represents a holistic approach to movement and perception and can help to promote people's independence and quality of life, especially in situations where there are movement restrictions or health challenges.

Laterality

Laterality refers to the dominance of one side of the body or a brain hemisphere in motor and sensory functions. The term is often used in connection with the preferred use of the right or left hand, leg, eyes, or ears. Here are some key aspects of laterality:

1. **Handedness:**
    - Handedness is an important aspect of laterality. The vast majority of people show a preference for using one hand for fine motor tasks. Most people are either right-handed or left-handed.
2. **Foot dominance:**
    - Similar to hand dominance, there is also a preference for using a specific foot for tasks such as climbing stairs or kicking a ball. Most people are right-footed or left-footed.
3. **Ocular dominance:**
    - Eye dominance refers to which eye is preferred for visual tasks. In most people, either the right or left eye dominates.
4. **Ear dominance:**
    - Ear dominance refers to the preferred use of an ear in auditory perception. People can be either right- or left-dominant in hearing.
5. **Hemisphere dominance:**
    - The brain hemispheres (right and left) are responsible for different functions. Hemisphere dominance refers to which side of the brain is preferred for certain cognitive or motor tasks. For example, the left hemisphere is often associated with language skills, while the right hemisphere may be responsible for spatial perception and creativity.
6. **Cross Dominance:**
    - In some people, there is cross-dominance, in which the hand preferred in writing does not align with the dominant side of the foot or eye.

Laterality often develops in the first years of life and can be influenced by genetic, but also environmental factors. Most people show a clear preference for the use of a particular side of the body, but there are also variations and mixed forms, especially in the area of cross-dominance.

Knowledge of laterality is important in various disciplines, including educational, therapeutic, and athletic settings, as it can influence the planning of interventions and activities.

Lifestyle

The rhythm of life refers to the recurring timing of events in a person's life. This rhythm is influenced by daily, seasonal and life phases and can vary individually. A stable rhythm of life can promote well-being, health, and productivity. The rhythm of life consists of:

1. **Circadian rhythm:**
    - The daily rhythm, also known as the circadian rhythm, refers to the natural sleep-wake cycle, which lasts about 24 hours. This rhythm is influenced by external factors such as light and darkness.
2. **Sleep Patterns:**
    - The regularity and quality of sleep are important elements of the rhythm of life. A good night's sleep is crucial for physical and mental health.
3. **Rhythm of work:**
    - The rhythm of work refers to the temporal structure of working hours, breaks and free time. A balanced work rhythm supports professional performance and well-being.
4. **Seasons and seasonal rhythms:**
    - The changes of the seasons affect the rhythm of life. People often adapt their activities, diet, and leisure activities to the different seasons.
5. **Stages:**
    - Different stages of life, such as childhood, adolescence, adulthood, and old age, have different demands and challenges that affect the rhythm of life.
6. **Rituals and habits:**
    - Personal rituals and habits, such as morning routines or evening relaxation rituals, can help maintain a stable rhythm of life.
7. **Social Interactions:**
    - The rhythm of social interactions, such as gatherings with friends or family gatherings, contributes to social well-being.

8. **Healthy nutrition:**
    - Regular meals and a balanced eating rhythm support health and energy levels.
9. **Exercise and physical activity:**
    - Incorporating regular exercise into the rhythm of life promotes physical fitness and well-being.
10. **Time management:**
    - Effective time management and organizing tasks in the rhythm of life can reduce stress and increase efficiency.

A balanced rhythm of life is important for overall well-being because it takes into account a person's biological, psychological, and social needs. Irregularities in the rhythm of life can lead to sleep disorders, stress and other health problems. However, it is important to note that the rhythm of life can be customized and can vary at different stages of life and circumstances.

Long-term memory

Long-term memory is a part of the human memory system that is responsible for the permanent storage of information. Unlike short-term memory, which is temporary and limited, long-term memory allows knowledge and experience to be retained for a longer period of time, possibly for life.

Here are some features and functions of long-term memory:

1. **Unlimited capacity:** Unlike limited short-term memory, long-term memory has an almost unlimited capacity for storing information.
2. **Long-lived storage:** Information that enters long-term memory can be stored for a longer period of time, even if it has initially passed through short-term memory.
3. **Organization of information:** Long-term memory organizes information in the form of structures of knowledge, including concepts, schemas, and connections between different pieces of information. This organization facilitates the access and retrieval of knowledge.
4. **Two main types:** Long-term memory is often divided into two main types:
    - **Explicit or declarative memory:** These are conscious memories of facts, events, and experiences. It can be further divided into episodic memory (events) and semantic memory (facts, concepts).
    - **Implicit or non-declarative memory:** This includes unconscious memories and skills, such as learning motor skills or emotional conditioning.
5. **Transfer from short-term to long-term memory:** Information usually passes through short-term memory before passing into long-term memory. Consolidation is the process by which information transitions from temporary to permanent memory.

Long-term memory plays a crucial role in identity, learning, problem-solving, and many other cognitive processes. It can be influenced by repeated learning, emotional connections, conscious attention, and other factors. In research and practice, various methods and techniques are used to understand and promote the formation and retrieval of information from long-term memory.

Low Vision

Low vision refers to a visual impairment in which a person has significant difficulty seeing, even when wearing optimally corrected glasses or contact lenses. Unlike blindness, a person with low vision retains some vision, but they are severely impaired. People with low vision may have difficulty reading, writing, recognizing faces, and navigating the environment. The causes of low vision can be many and include eye diseases, injuries, or genetic factors.

Here are some points related to Low Vision:

1. **Impaired visual acuity:**
   - People with low vision have reduced visual acuity. This means that they can see objects out of focus or blurry, even if they are close to the eyes.
2. **Scotoma:**
   - Some people with low vision may have problems with the visual field. This means that they may have difficulty seeing objects in their lateral or peripheral field of vision.
3. **Glare sensitivity:**
   - Many people with low vision are more sensitive to bright light and glare, which can further affect their vision.
4. **Contrast Sensitivity:**
   - Contrasts between objects can be difficult for people with low vision to see. This is especially true for the difference between dark and light areas.
5. **Difficulty reading:**
   - Reading can be very challenging. People with low vision may have difficulty recognizing letters or words, even with the greatest effort.
6. **Limited independence:**
   - Impaired vision can affect independence by making everyday activities such as shopping, cooking, or recognizing road signs more difficult.

7. **Tools and Technologies:**
    - There are various tools and technologies that can support people with low vision. These include magnifying glasses, screen readers, voice-controlled devices, and other adaptive technologies.
8. **Rehabilitation Training:**
    - People with low vision can benefit from rehabilitation training, where they learn to use adaptive strategies to better manage their daily lives.

Low vision can vary from person to person, and the impact on daily life can vary depending on a person's specific vision problems. Early diagnosis, professional support from ophthalmologists and rehabilitation professionals, and the use of aids and technologies can help improve the quality of life of people with low vision.

Lymphatic drainage

Lymphatic drainage is a therapeutic technique that aims to promote the movement of lymph in the lymphatic system. The lymphatic system is a part of the immune system and plays an important role in removing waste, toxins, and excess fluid from the body's tissues. Lymphatic drainage is performed by specially trained therapists and can be used for various medical conditions. Here is some more information about lymphatic drainage:

1. **Manual Techniques:**
   - Lymphatic drainage is usually performed manually, with the therapist applying gentle, rhythmic movements and pressure to the skin. This helps to stimulate the lymphatic vessels and promote drainage.
2. **Promotion of lymphatic circulation:**
   - The aim is to support the natural circulation of lymph and reduce congestion or accumulation of lymphatic fluid.
3. **Reduction of edema:**
   - Lymphatic drainage is often used for edema (swelling), whether due to lymphedema, postoperative swelling, or other causes.
4. **Postoperative use:**
   - After certain surgical procedures, especially in the area of the lymph nodes, lymphatic drainage can help minimize postoperative swelling and promote recovery.
5. **Detoxification and relaxation:**
   - Although the primary function of lymphatic drainage is to improve lymphatic flow, it is also sometimes used for detoxification and relaxation.
6. **Use for lymphedema:**
   - People who suffer from primary or secondary lymphedema may benefit from regular lymphatic drainage sessions to alleviate discomfort and improve quality of life.

7. **Indications for certain clinical pictures:**
    - Lymphatic drainage can also be used for various conditions such as venous diseases, rheumatic diseases and inflammations.
8. **Specialized Training:**
    - Therapists who perform lymphatic drainage have undergone specialized training to use the right techniques and measures.

Lymphatic drainage should only be performed by trained professionals, as improper applications or too much pressure can damage the lymphatic system. The technique is often used as part of a comprehensive therapeutic approach, which can vary depending on individual needs and health status.

Manual Therapy

Manual therapy is a physiotherapeutic treatment method that focuses on the examination and treatment of functional disorders of the musculoskeletal system. The aim is to relieve pain, improve mobility and optimize the function of joints and muscles. This form of therapy is carried out by specially trained professionals, such as physiotherapists or osteopaths. Here are some important features of manual therapy:

1. **Manual Examination:**
   - The therapist will perform a thorough manual examination to identify dysfunction, limitations in mobility, and painful areas in the musculoskeletal system.
2. **Joint mobilization:**
   - Through gentle movements and mobilization techniques, the therapist tries to restore normal joint mobility. This can help reduce stiffness and improve flexibility.
3. **Manipulation Techniques:**
   - In some cases, manipulation techniques may be used, in which the therapist makes quick, controlled movements on a joint to improve mobility. This is often referred to as "joint manipulation" or "manipulation."
4. **Soft Tissue Techniques:**
   - The therapist may also use special techniques to release tension and adhesions in the muscles and surrounding tissues. These include massages, stretching, and trigger point therapy.
5. **Patient counseling and exercises:**
   - Part of the manual therapy is also patient counseling. The therapist can recommend exercises and self-help measures to the patient to support and maintain treatment results in the long term.

6. **Indications:**
   - Manual therapy can be used for various musculoskeletal problems, including back pain, neck pain, joint pain, osteoarthritis and other functional impairments.
7. **Individualized therapy plans:**
   - The application of manual therapy is individual, based on the specific diagnosis and needs of the individual patient. The therapy plan is adapted to the personal anatomy and state of health.
8. **Training and Certification:**
   - Therapists who use manual therapy have undergone special training and further education. The application of these techniques requires a deep understanding of anatomy, biomechanics and pathophysiology.

Manual therapy should only be performed by well-trained and licensed professionals. The selection of techniques and their application should be based on an accurate diagnosis and individual needs. Manual therapy can be an effective adjunct to other physical therapy approaches and is often used as part of a comprehensive rehabilitation program.

Material Adaptation

Material adaptation refers to the adaptation of materials or resources to meet the individual needs of people with special requirements. This approach is relevant in various fields, including education, healthcare, rehabilitation, and inclusion. Material adaptations can help improve accessibility, use, and participation for people with different abilities or needs. Here are some examples and contexts in which material adaptation can be applied:

1. **Education:**
    - In schools, materials, textbooks, or classroom resources can be adapted to meet the needs of students with learning disabilities or physical impairments. This may include the use of larger fonts, audiovisual aids, or tactile materials.
2. **Health service:**
    - In healthcare, patient information, guidance or rehabilitation materials can be adapted to the specific needs of people with different health conditions. This could include the use of easy-to-understand languages, visual aids, or specialized equipment.
3. **Rehabilitation:**
    - In rehabilitation, materials used for therapeutic exercises or activities can be adapted to take into account patients' individual abilities and limitations. This could include the use of specialized aids, modified tools, or customized training programs.
4. **Workplace:**
    - In the workplace, materials, work equipment or software solutions can be adapted to the needs of employees with disabilities to improve accessibility and promote job performance.
5. **Technology:**
    - In technology, software applications, apps, or electronic devices can be adapted to the needs of people with different abilities. This may include the

integration of voice control, screen enlargements, or other accessible features.

6. **Communication:**
   - For people with communication disorders, assisted communication materials, such as pictorial symbols, sign language, or special writing aids, can be adapted to facilitate effective communication.

7. **Leisure and culture:**
   - In leisure and cultural areas, events, games or cultural materials can be adapted to allow people with different needs to participate. This could include providing audio descriptions in theatrical performances or adapting games for people with motor impairments.

Material adaptation is an important aspect of inclusive design and aims to ensure that all people, regardless of their abilities or limitations, have equal access to information, education, health care and other resources.

Medication Management

Medication management refers to the safe and effective administration of medications to ensure optimal health and therapy outcomes for the patient. This process involves various aspects, from prescribing and obtaining medications, to taking them correctly, to monitoring side effects and interactions. Effective medication management is critical to maximizing therapeutic efficacy and minimizing the risk of complications. Medication Management Points:

1. **Prescription and diagnosis:**
   - The process begins with the correct diagnosis and prescription of medications by qualified medical professionals. This requires a comprehensive knowledge of the patient's history, symptoms, and appropriate medical interventions.
2. **Medication procurement:**
   - Patients need to make sure they are getting their medications from trusted sources, whether it's pharmacies or other approved providers.
3. **Instructions for use:**
   - Patients should strictly follow the instructions given by the doctor or pharmacist. This includes dosage, frequency, and duration of medication use.
4. **Drug interactions:**
   - Patients should tell their doctor or pharmacist about any medications, supplements, or herbal preparations they are taking to avoid potential interactions.
5. **Side effects and reactions:**
   - It is important to be aware of possible side effects or adverse reactions to medications and to report them to the healthcare professional. This allows for timely adjustment of therapy if necessary.
6. **Medication Schedule:**
   - Creating a medication schedule can help keep track of medications to take, dosages, and times. This is

especially important if several medications are taken at the same time.
7. **Patient education:**
   - Comprehensive patient education about their medications, including effects, side effects, and correct use, is crucial. This should be done in a language that is understandable to the patient.
8. **Self-management:**
   - Patients can be empowered to self-manage their medication management through training and support, especially for chronic conditions that require long-term medication use.
9. **Monitoring and Adjustment:**
   - Doctors regularly monitor the effectiveness of the prescribed medication, adjust the dosage if necessary, and take into account changes in the patient's state of health.

Effective medication management is critical to ensuring that patients get the best possible outcomes from their therapy, while also remaining safe and free of unnecessary risks. It requires close collaboration between patients, healthcare professionals and pharmacists.

Mentalization

Mentalization refers to the ability to understand other people's thoughts, intentions, feelings, and motivations and to recognize oneself as a thinking individual. It is a cognitive process that makes it possible to recognize and interpret the inner states of oneself and others. Mentalization plays a crucial role in social interactions, interpersonal relationships, and the regulation of emotions. Mentalization includes:

1. **Theory of Mind:**
    - Mentalization is closely related to the "Theory of Mind" (ToM), a term from psychology that describes the ability to put oneself in other people's perspective and understand their thoughts and feelings.
2. **Self-reflection:**
    - In addition to perceiving the thoughts of others, mentalization also includes the ability for self-reflection, in which one can understand one's own thoughts and feelings and place them in a larger context.
3. **Empathy:**
    - Mentalization is an important component of empathy. It allows you to put yourself in the shoes of others and resonate with their emotions.
4. **Social Interaction:**
    - In social interactions, mentalization is crucial for understanding other people's intentions, motivations, and emotions. It helps reduce misunderstandings and promote effective communication.
5. **Development process:**
    - The ability to mentalize develops over the course of childhood and adolescence. It is closely linked to the developing Theory of Mind and plays a role in the formation of secure attachments and social skills.

6. **Mentalization-Based Therapy (MBT):**
    - In psychiatry and psychotherapy, mentalization-based therapy is used as an approach to support people with mentalization disorders, such as borderline personality disorder. The development of the ability to mentalize is the focus of the therapeutic intervention.
7. **Emotion Regulation:**
    - Through the ability to mentalize, people can better understand and regulate their own emotions. This is especially important for dealing with stress, conflict, and other emotionally stressful situations.
8. **Cultural differences:**
    - Cultural differences can affect the way people mentalize. Different cultural backgrounds can bring different perspectives and interpretations of emotions and social cues.

Mentalization plays a fundamental role in our social world and helps to develop effective interpersonal relationships. An adequate understanding of the thoughts and feelings of oneself and others is crucial for developing and maintaining healthy social bonds.

Mirror Therapy

Mirror therapy is a therapeutic technique used in the rehabilitation of people with neurological or orthopedic problems. It is widely used in the treatment of phantom limbs after amputations, complex regional pain syndromes (CRPS), strokes, and other diseases of the neuromuscular system. The basic idea of mirror therapy is to use visual feedback to deceive the brain and improve the perception and function of limbs.

Here are the basic principles and applications of mirror therapy:

1. **Structure and arrangement:** The patient sits or stands in such a way that he has a mirror in front of him. For example, if the left upper limb is affected, the mirror is placed to make the right upper limb visible as if the left were present.
2. **Observing movements:** The patient then performs movements with the healthy (visible) limb while at the same time seeing the image of the healthy limb in the mirror. The brain interprets this as movement of the affected limb.
3. **Brain deception:** The visual feedback from the mirror deceives the brain by making it feel that the affected limb is functioning normally. This can help improve sensory perception and motor function.
4. **Pain relief:** In patients with complex regional pain syndromes (CRPS), mirror therapy can help reduce pain by stimulating the brain in a positive way.
5. **Use for phantom limbs:** In people with amputations, mirror therapy can be used to relieve the sensation of a phantom limb. The patient sees the intact limb in the mirror and can move it, which stimulates the brain to "feel" the lost limb.
6. **Training and recovery:** Mirror therapy is often used as part of a broader rehabilitation program to improve mobility, coordination, and functionality of the affected limb.

Mirror therapy is a method based on the brain's ability to process visual feedback and influence motor functions.

Motor

Motor function refers to the body's ability to plan, coordinate, and execute movements. It is a comprehensive concept that encompasses both gross motor skills (such as walking, running, and jumping) and fine motor skills (such as grasping, writing, and manipulating small objects). Motor skills are crucial for participation in everyday activities and influence physical health, well-being and social integration.

Motor skills can be divided into two main categories:

1. **Gross motor skills:** This refers to the ability to coordinate larger muscle groups to perform movements such as walking, running, jumping, throwing, or catching. Gross motor skills are important for locomotion and participation in sports activities.
2. **Fine motor skills:** This refers to the precision and coordination of small muscles, especially the hands and fingers. Fine motor skills are crucial for tasks such as writing, drawing, closing buttons, using cutlery, and other activities that require precise hand-eye coordination.

The development of motor skills occurs at different stages during childhood, starting with basic reflexes in infancy and ending with more complex motor skills in adolescence. Motor skills can be influenced by genetic factors, environmental stimuli, physical activity, and experience.

Some people may experience motor skills challenges due to genetic conditions, developmental disorders, or injuries. In these cases, targeted occupational therapy or physiotherapy intervention can help improve motor skills and promote quality of life.

However, motor skills remain a lifelong process that can be supported by regular physical activity and training even in adulthood. Good motor skills are important not only for physical health, but also for psychosocial development and coping with everyday life.

Motorized planning

Motor planning refers to the cognitive process in which the brain plans, organizes, and prepares the control and coordination of movements. This process is crucial for the execution of motor actions and includes various cognitive and sensory aspects to allow effective and precise movement.

Points of motor planning are:

1. **Goal setting:** Motor planning begins with setting a clear goal or intention for the planned movement. This can range from simple actions such as grasping an object to more complex activities such as playing an instrument.
2. **Sensory information processing:** The brain processes sensory information from various sources, including visual perception, proprioceptive information (such as the position of the limbs in space), and tactile information.
3. **Choice of movement strategy:** Based on the target and the available sensory information, the brain selects an appropriate movement strategy. This may include selecting specific muscles, joint angles, and movement patterns.
4. **Temporal organization:** Motor planning also includes the temporal organization of movement, including the coordination of muscles and joints to ensure fluid and precise execution.
5. **Adaptation to changes:** During the execution of a movement, there may be unexpected changes in the environment or in the body. Motor planning allows adaptation to such changes in real time to maintain control over movement.

Motor planning is involved in various parts of the nervous system, including the motor cortex in the brain, the basal ganglia, and the cerebellum. Disorders in motor planning can lead to movement restrictions, coordination problems and other motor deficits.

In rehabilitation and therapeutic practice, targeted exercises and interventions are often used to improve motor planning, especially in individuals with neurological disorders or injuries.

Multimodal Therapy

Multimodal therapy is an integrative approach to therapy that combines multiple therapeutic methods and interventions to meet a patient's individual needs. This approach takes into account that different people respond differently to different therapies and that a combination of different approaches is often more effective than a single method. Multimodal therapy is applied in various areas of health care, including psychiatry, pain management, rehabilitation, and other medical disciplines. Here are some key aspects of multimodal therapy:

1. **Integration of different forms of therapy:**
   - Multimodal therapy integrates various therapeutic modalities, including drug treatment, psychotherapy, cognitive behavioral therapy, physical therapy, occupational therapy, and other appropriate approaches.
2. **Individualization of the treatment:**
   - The selection of therapeutic approaches is adapted to the individual needs, diagnosis and specific challenges of the patient. The therapy is individually adapted.
3. **Holistic approach:**
   - The multimodal approach takes into account the different aspects of well-being, including physical, psychological and social dimensions. The therapy aims to support the patient holistically.
4. **Treatment of comorbidities:**
   - Patients with multiple concurrent health problems or mental disorders may benefit from multimodal therapy, which aims to treat multiple aspects of their health at the same time.
5. **Pain management:**
   - In pain management, multimodal therapy is often used to manage pain in a variety of ways, including drug approaches, physical therapy, psychological support, and non-drug strategies.

6. **Psychiatric treatment:**
   - For psychiatric disorders, multimodal therapy can combine medication, psychotherapy, behavioral interventions, and other therapeutic elements to provide comprehensive treatment.
7. **Addiction Treatment:**
   - In addiction therapy, multimodal therapy can combine different approaches such as drug weaning, cognitive behavioral therapy, support groups, and other interventions.
8. **Rehabilitation:**
   - In rehabilitation after injuries or surgeries, multimodal therapy can combine different forms of therapy to support recovery and the restoration of functionality.

Multimodal therapy requires close collaboration between different professionals, including doctors, therapists, nurses, and other healthcare providers. The integration of different therapeutic approaches enables comprehensive care and takes into account the complexity of health conditions and individual needs.

Music therapy

Music therapy is a cross-disciplinary form of therapy that uses music as a central element in promoting physical, emotional, cognitive, and social health and well-being. A trained music therapist uses musical activities to achieve therapeutic goals and address individual needs. Music therapy can be used in a variety of contexts, including clinical work, educational institutions, nursing homes, and psychosocial support programs. Music therapy includes:

1. **Customization:**
   - Music therapy can be individually adapted to the needs of each individual. It can benefit people of all ages, from children to seniors.
2. **Clinical Applications:**
   - In clinical practice, music therapy is used to treat people with various health conditions, including mental illnesses, neurological disorders, developmental disorders, trauma, and others.
3. **Different modalities:**
   - Music therapy can include various modalities, including active music-making, listening to music, singing, songwriting, movement to music, and improvisation.
4. **Promoting expression and communication:**
   - Music provides a creative platform for expressing feelings and thoughts, especially for people who have difficulty expressing themselves verbally.
5. **Emotion Regulation:**
   - Music therapy can help recognize, understand, and regulate emotions. Music can provide a non-verbal way to process emotions.
6. **Cognitive stimulation:**
   - In the treatment of neurological diseases, such as Alzheimer's or other dementias, music therapy can stimulate cognitive function and have positive effects on memory and attention.
7. **Social Interaction:**

- Group music therapy can promote social interaction by supporting group collaboration through making music together and creating creatively.

8. **Relaxation and stress relief:**
    - Music can serve as a means of relaxation and stress management. Slow, soothing melodies can have a relaxing effect.
9. **Motor rehabilitation:**
    - In rehabilitation after injuries or strokes, music therapy can be used to improve motor skills and coordination.
10. **Evaluation and documentation:**
    - Music therapists conduct assessments to monitor progress and document the effectiveness of interventions.

Music therapy is based on the idea that the structured and creative elements of music can have a positive impact on physical and mental health. By integrating music into the therapeutic process, individual goals can be achieved and quality of life can be improved.

Neurology

Neurology is a medical specialty that specializes in the diagnosis and treatment of diseases of the nervous system. The nervous system includes the brain, spinal cord, peripheral nerves, and muscles. Neurologists are medical specialists who specialize in the examination, diagnosis, and treatment of conditions such as stroke, epilepsy, headaches, dementia, multiple sclerosis, Parkinson's disease, and many other neurological disorders. Points of neurology:

1. **Brain and spinal cord:**
    - Neurology deals with diseases of the central nervous system, which includes the brain and spinal cord. This includes neurological diseases, injuries and degenerative processes.
2. **Peripheral nerves:**
    - In addition to the central nervous system, neurology also takes care of diseases of the peripheral nerves, which transmit signals between the central nervous system and the muscles and other organs.
3. **Neurological examinations:**
    - Neurologists use various diagnostic procedures to identify neurological disorders. These include clinical examinations, imaging techniques such as CT or MRI scans, electroencephalography (EEG) to measure brain activity, and other tests.
4. **Stroke Treatment:**
    - Neurologists play a crucial role in the treatment of stroke, an acute condition caused by impaired blood supply to the brain. Early intervention is crucial to minimize the consequences of a stroke.
5. **Epilepsy Treatment:**
    - Epilepsy is a neurological disorder that leads to recurrent seizures. Neurologists are involved in the diagnosis and management of epilepsy, often using anticonvulsant medications.
6. **Movement disorders:**

- Neurologists also treat conditions associated with disorders of movement and coordination, including Parkinson's disease, tremor, chorea, and dystonia.

7. **Multiple Sclerosis (MS):**
   - MS is an autoimmune disease that affects the central nervous system. Neurologists are involved in the diagnosis and treatment of MS, including the administration of immunomodulators.

8. **Headache and migraine:**
   - Neurologists also treat headaches and migraines by identifying the causes and suggesting appropriate therapies.

9. **Neurorehabilitation:**
   - After neurological events or surgery, neurorehabilitation may be necessary to restore or improve functions. This may include physical therapy, occupational therapy, and speech therapy.

Neurology is a broad field that is constantly evolving. Advances in imaging, neuroscience, and treatment options have helped improve the diagnosis and treatment of neurological disorders. Collaboration with other medical specialties, such as neurosurgery, psychiatry, and rehabilitation, is often integral to providing comprehensive care for patients with neurological disorders.

Neuropsychological Rehabilitation

Neuropsychological rehabilitation is a specialized area of rehabilitation that aims to help people with neurological diseases or injuries improve, compensate, or relearn their cognitive functions. This process is designed to increase the quality of life of those affected and to restore or maximize their abilities in everyday activities. Here is some information about neuropsychological rehabilitation:

1. **Diagnostics and evaluation:**
    - Rehabilitation often begins with a comprehensive neuropsychological diagnosis to understand the nature and extent of cognitive impairment. This includes tests and assessments of memory, attention, executive function, and other cognitive areas.
2. **Individual objectives:**
    - Based on the diagnostic results, individual rehabilitation goals are set based on the specific needs and abilities of the affected person.
3. **Cognitive Exercises and Therapy:**
    - Neuropsychological rehabilitation often includes cognitive exercises and therapies aimed at improving cognitive function. This may include memory training, problem-solving strategies, attentional exercises, and other cognitive interventions.
4. **Compensation techniques:**
    - People with neurological impairments can learn compensatory techniques to better deal with their cognitive challenges. This includes information organization strategies, time management, and other tools.
5. **Exercises relevant to everyday life:**
    - Neuropsychological rehabilitation often emphasizes the practice of the acquired skills in situations relevant to everyday life. This may include shopping, cooking, traveling, or other daily activities.
6. **Family and family involvement:**

- The involvement of family members and caregivers is often integral to the success of rehabilitation. Training and support for loved ones can help create a supportive environment.
7. **Emotional Support:**
    - Neurological impairments can present emotional challenges. Neuropsychological rehabilitation may also include emotional support and counseling to deal with the psychological effects of the impairments.
8. **Long-term support and monitoring:**
    - Rehabilitation is often a long-term process. After formal rehabilitation is complete, long-term care and monitoring may be necessary to ensure that progress is maintained and quality of life improves.

Neuropsychological rehabilitation is of great importance for people with acquired brain damage, strokes, traumatic brain injuries or neurodegenerative diseases. It requires interdisciplinary collaboration between neuropsychologists, physiotherapists, occupational therapists, speech therapists and other professionals to ensure comprehensive and effective rehabilitation.

Neuropsychology

Neuropsychology is a branch of psychology that deals with the study of the relationship between brain function and behavior. It combines principles of psychology with knowledge of the anatomical and physiological properties of the brain. Neuropsychologists study how different brain regions and structures are related to cognitive, emotional, and behavioral functions. Further information from Neuropsychology:

1. **Brain Functions:**
   - Neuropsychology studies how specific brain functions influence behavior. These include cognitive functions such as attention, memory, language, perception, thinking, and emotional regulation.
2. **Brain damage and disorders:**
   - Neuropsychologists study the effects of brain damage, neurological disorders, or genetic factors on cognitive and emotional function. This also includes psychiatric disorders with a neurobiological basis.
3. **Diagnostics:**
   - Neuropsychologists use standardized tests and clinical assessments to identify cognitive deficits and understand patterns of brain damage. These diagnostic procedures can help in the planning of interventions and the development of treatment plans.
4. **Rehabilitation:**
   - In neuropsychology, rehabilitation plays an important role in helping people with brain damage or disorders recover, adapt, and improve their cognitive abilities.
5. **Research:**
   - Neuropsychologists participate in research to deepen the understanding of brain-behavioral relationships. This can include both experimental studies and clinical research.

6. **Developmental Neuropsychology:**
   - This area studies the development of cognitive functions throughout life and how the developing brain affects behavior.
7. **Cognitive Neuroscience:**
   - Cognitive neuroscience is an interdisciplinary perspective that combines insights from neuropsychology, psychology, and neuroscience to understand the interplay between the brain and cognition.
8. **Clinical Application:**
   - In clinical application, neuropsychology offers insights into the diagnosis and treatment of conditions such as stroke, trauma, neurodegenerative diseases, epilepsy, and psychiatric disorders.
9. **Neuropsychological Therapy:**
   - Based on the findings of neuropsychology, individualized therapeutic interventions are developed to improve or compensate for cognitive functions.
10. **Advice and support:**
    - Neuropsychologists often offer counseling and support to patients and their families to help them navigate challenges related to cognitive impairment.

Neuropsychology plays a key role in integrating knowledge about the structure and function of the brain into psychological research and practice. It has far-reaching implications for the diagnosis and treatment of people with neurological or psychological disorders.

Nystagmus

Nystagmus is an involuntary, rhythmic movement of the eyes that can have various causes. This eye movement is characterized by fast phases in one direction and slower, opposite phases in the other. Nystagmus can be horizontal, vertical or oblique.

There are different types of nystagmus, and the manifestations can vary depending on the cause and situation. Some of the main types of nystagmus include:

1. **Physiological nystagmus:** This is the normal, physiological nystagmus that occurs in certain situations, such as turning your head rapidly or when you are extremely tired.
2. **Pathological nystagmus:** This occurs due to disorders in the visual system, vestibular system (ear) or central nervous system. It can indicate neurological disorders, developmental disorders, or other health problems.
3. **Conjugated nystagmus:** In this case, both eyes move in the same direction at the same time.
4. **Disconjugated nystagmus:** In this form, the eyes move independently of each other.
5. **Manifested and latent:** Nystagmus can be manifest (obvious) or latent (hidden). A latent nystagmus usually only becomes visible with a certain eye movement or direction of gaze.

The causes of nystagmus can be varied. They range from congenital disorders and neurological disorders to certain medications or toxin exposures. An accurate diagnosis often requires a comprehensive examination by an ophthalmologist or neurologist.

Treatment for nystagmus depends on the underlying cause. In some cases, treatment may be aimed at relieving symptoms or treating the underlying condition. In other cases, such as congenital nystagmus, the goal may be to improve quality of life and support functionality in everyday life.

Orthopaedic technology

Orthopaedic technology is a field that deals with the development, manufacture and adaptation of orthopaedic aids and technical solutions for people with limited mobility. The aim is to improve the quality of life and mobility of people with orthopaedic impairments. Key aspects of orthopaedic technology:

1. **Prostheses:**
   - Prosthetists design, manufacture, and fit prostheses to replace lost or amputated limbs. The goal is to achieve optimal functionality and aesthetics.
2. **Orthotics:**
   - Orthotics are orthopedic aids that are placed on the body to support, stabilize, or correct joints. Orthopaedic technicians develop individual orthoses that are tailored to the specific needs of the patient.
3. **Orthopedic shoe insoles:**
   - Another area of orthopedic technology includes the production of custom-made orthopedic shoe insoles, which are used to correct foot problems, distribute pressure and improve gait mechanics.
4. **Wheelchairs and walking aids:**
   - Prosthetists are also involved in the fitting of wheelchairs and walking aids. This can include the selection of suitable models, the adjustment of seating positions and the integration of special functions.
5. **Adapted vehicles:**
   - In some cases, orthopaedic technology may also include the adaptation of vehicles for people with mobility impairments to make it easier for them to move around independently.
6. **Technological innovations:**
   - Advances in orthopedic technology also include technological innovations, such as the integration of robotics, sensors, and artificial intelligence to improve the functionality of prostheses and orthotics.

7. **Customization and customization:**
   - A central aspect of orthopaedic technology is the individualisation and adaptation of the aids to the specific anatomical and functional requirements of each individual.
8. **Rehabilitation support:**
   - Prosthetists often work closely with physical therapists and physicians to ensure that orthopedic aids optimally support the rehabilitation process.
9. **Patient counselling and training:**
   - Prosthetists often provide patient counseling and training to ensure that assistive devices are used effectively and patient needs are met.
10. **Quality Control and Research:**
    - Orthopedic technology also includes quality control procedures to ensure that the aids manufactured meet the required standards. Research in this area aims to drive continuous improvement and innovation.

Orthopedic technology plays a crucial role in the rehabilitation and support of people with orthopedic challenges. By combining craftsmanship, technological innovation and customization, prosthetists can help improve the quality of life and independence of people with limited mobility.

Orthopaedics

Orthopedics is a medical specialty specializing in the diagnosis, treatment, prevention, and rehabilitation of diseases and injuries of the musculoskeletal system. The musculoskeletal system includes bones, joints, muscles, tendons, ligaments, and other structures associated with the musculoskeletal system. Orthopedic surgeons are specialists who specialize in the care of patients with diseases of the musculoskeletal system. Further information from the orthopaedics:

1. **Diagnosis and Imaging:**
    - Orthopedic surgeons use clinical examinations, imaging techniques such as X-rays, CT scans, and MRI, as well as laboratory tests to diagnose orthopedic conditions.
2. **Fracture Treatment:**
    - Orthopaedic surgeons specialise in the treatment of bone fractures and can perform conservative measures such as plaster casts or surgical interventions such as fixations.
3. **Joint Replacement Surgery:**
    - In cases of advanced joint diseases, such as osteoarthritis, orthopedic surgeons can perform joint replacement surgery, such as hip or knee arthroplasty.
4. **Arthroscopy:**
    - Orthopedics also includes arthroscopic procedures, in which small instruments are inserted into the joint through tiny incisions to perform diagnostic or therapeutic procedures.
5. **Sports medicine:**
    - Orthopedic surgeons often work in the field of sports medicine to treat sports injuries, recommend preventive measures, and guide rehabilitation after injuries.

6. **Spine Surgery:**
   - Orthopedic surgeons can also treat spinal disorders and injuries, including intervertebral disc problems, vertebral fractures, and spinal deformities.
7. **Conservative therapy:**
   - In addition to surgical procedures, orthopedic surgeons also offer conservative therapy options, including physical therapy, medications, orthopedic aids, and injections.
8. **Paediatric orthopaedics:**
   - Pediatric orthopedic surgeons specialize in the treatment of orthopedic conditions in children, including congenital malformations and developmental disorders.
9. **Rheumatological diseases:**
   - Orthopedic surgeons can also play a role in rheumatological diseases, such as rheumatoid arthritis or gout, in collaboration with rheumatologists.
10. **Prevention and rehabilitation:**
    - Orthopaedic surgeons are involved in preventive measures to prevent injuries and diseases of the musculoskeletal system. They also play a key role in rehabilitation after orthopedic procedures or injuries.

Orthopedics is a versatile specialty that treats a wide range of diseases and injuries affecting the musculoskeletal system. Modern orthopedics integrates advanced diagnostic technologies, minimally invasive surgery, conservative therapeutic approaches, and comprehensive rehabilitation to provide the best possible care for patients with orthopedic challenges.

OTIPM Model

The Occupational Therapy Intervention Process Model (OTIPM) is a model in occupational therapy that structures and guides the intervention process. It was developed by Mary Law, Sue Baptiste and Anne Carswell and is based on the Canadian Model of Occupational Performance (CMOP).

The OTIPM consists of six main phases that describe the process of occupational therapy intervention:

1. **Reflection and Information Gathering:** In this phase, information about the client is collected, including their individual characteristics, values, interests, and life situation. The occupational therapist also reflects on his own assumptions and values.
2. **Goal Setting:** Based on the information collected, goals are set together with the client. These goals are aimed at improving the client's ability to act and participate in his or her life context.
3. **Planning:** The occupational therapist develops an intervention plan that outlines the specific actions and interventions to be taken to achieve the set goals. This plan takes into account the client's resources as well as the context of their environment.
4. **Implementation:** In this phase, the planned interventions are implemented. The occupational therapist works directly with the client to achieve the identified goals. This can include both individual and group-based interventions.
5. **Monitoring:** The progress of the intervention is monitored to ensure that the strategies chosen are effective. Adjustments can be made if necessary, and progress is continuously assessed.
6. **Assessment and Evaluation:** At the end of the intervention process, a comprehensive assessment of the objectives achieved and the overall progress is made. The occupational therapist and the client reflect together on the intervention process and discuss the next steps.

The OTIPM is an action-guiding model that supports occupational therapists in adopting a systematic and customer-centric approach to the planning and implementation of their interventions. It emphasizes the importance of collaboration between the occupational therapist and the client throughout the process.

Pain Management

Pain management refers to the application of strategies and interventions to alleviate pain, minimize its effects, and improve the quality of life of individuals with pain. Pain can have many causes, from acute injuries to chronic conditions, and pain management aims to use individualized approaches to reduce pain to a tolerable level. Here are some features of pain management:

1. **Multidisciplinary approach:**
    - Effective pain management often involves a multidisciplinary approach that involves different professionals working together. These can include doctors, pain management professionals, physical therapists, psychologists, and other health care providers.
2. **Pain Rating:**
    - A comprehensive pain assessment is the starting point for effective pain management. It assesses the type, intensity, duration and effects of the pain in order to create an individualized treatment plan.
3. **Drug therapy:**
    - Drug approaches may include painkillers, anti-inflammatory drugs, muscle relaxants, and other medications. The choice of medication depends on the type of pain and individual factors.
4. **Physiotherapy and rehabilitation:**
    - Physical therapy can help improve functionality, correct muscle imbalances, and promote mobility. Rehabilitation may also include targeted exercises and techniques for pain relief.
5. **Psychological support:**
    - Psychological interventions, such as cognitive behavioral therapy, can help change attitudes toward pain, manage stress, and improve pain management.

6. **Interventional procedures:**
   - For certain pain conditions, interventional procedures such as injections, nerve blocks, or neurostimulation can be used to relieve the pain.
7. **Alternative therapies:**
   - Some people find relief through alternative therapies such as acupuncture, massage, yoga, or relaxation techniques. These can be used as part of a comprehensive pain management plan.
8. **Lifestyle Modifications:**
   - Lifestyle changes, including regular exercise, a healthy diet, adequate sleep, and stress management, can have a positive impact on pain management.
9. **Patient education and self-management:**
   - Educating the patient about the pain, its causes, and coping strategies is crucial. Patients should be involved in care and learn how to manage their pain themselves.
10. **Long-term care and aftercare:**
    - Chronic pain often requires long-term care and aftercare. Continuing care and adjusting the treatment plan are important to achieve sustainable pain relief.

Optimal pain management should be individualized, as pain is a complex and subjective experience. Cooperation with experts from various disciplines enables comprehensive and targeted support.

Painting Therapy

Painting therapy is a form of creative therapy that uses painting as a means of self-expression, self-discovery, and therapeutic change. This form of therapy can be performed by professionals such as art therapists or psychotherapists and is designed to help people express their emotions, reduce stress, boost their creativity, and overcome personal challenges. Further information on painting therapy:

1. **Self-expression:**
   - Painting therapy allows clients to express their feelings, thoughts, and experiences in a non-verbal way. Creating and shaping can serve as a language that goes beyond words.
2. **Self-discovery:**
   - Through creative creation during painting therapy, people can delve deeper into their own emotions and inner processes, which can lead to self-discovery and self-knowledge.
3. **Stress:**
   - Painting can be a relaxing and stress-reducing activity. It allows clients to focus on the creative process and temporarily disconnect from stressful thoughts and feelings.
4. **Fostering creativity:**
   - Painting therapy can nurture a person's creative side and help develop innovative ways of thinking and solutions.
5. **Communication without words:**
   - Especially for people who have difficulty expressing their feelings in words, painting therapy offers an alternative form of communication.
6. **Coping with Trauma:**
   - For people who have experienced trauma, painting therapy can help process and express unexpressed emotions.

7. **Group or individual therapy:**
    - Painting therapy can be done in both individual and group sessions. In the group, creative exchange and shared experience can be supportive.
8. **Integration into psychotherapeutic approaches:**
    - Maltherapy can be used in conjunction with other psychotherapeutic approaches and can serve as an integral part of a comprehensive therapy plan.
9. **Materials and techniques:**
    - In painting therapy, various materials such as paints, brushes, chalks, paper or canvases are used. The choice of materials and techniques may vary depending on the client's needs and preferences.

Painting therapy can be used in a variety of settings, including mental health care, rehabilitation, palliative care, addiction therapy, and more.

In painting therapy, in which the creative process is in the foreground, there is no "right" or "wrong" in the traditional sense. It's about using the experience to promote personal growth and well-being.

Palliative care

Palliative care is an approach in medical care that aims to improve the quality of life of patients suffering from severe, often progressive or life-threatening illnesses. The focus is on alleviating pain, other symptoms, and psychosocial and spiritual well-being. Palliative care can be provided in a variety of settings, including hospitals, care facilities, or in the home setting. Palliative care includes:

1. **Holistic approach:**
   - Palliative care looks at the patient as a whole, including their physical, psychological, social, and spiritual needs. The holistic approach aims to take into account all aspects of the patient and their quality of life.
2. **Pain & Symptom Control:**
   - Palliative care deals intensively with the control of pain and other distressing symptoms. This may include the use of medications, physical therapies, and alternative approaches.
3. **Psycho-social support:**
   - Palliative care also includes supporting the psychosocial needs of patients and their families. This includes emotional support, counseling, communication about disease progression, and help with care-related decisions.
4. **Spiritual Care:**
   - Spiritual care is an essential part of palliative care. It respects individual belief systems and provides support for spiritual needs and questions.
5. **Communication and decision-making:**
   - Palliative care emphasizes open and honest communication between patients, families, and the care team. This includes the discussion of treatment options, quality of life and end-of-life decisions.
6. **End-of-life care:**
   - Palliative care also includes the care of patients at the end of life. This includes respect for the patient's

wishes, pain management, emotional support, and family support.

7. **Hospice Care:**
   - In some cases, palliative care may be related to hospice care. Hospice care focuses on caring for people in the final stages of their lives, providing comprehensive support for patients and their families.

8. **Involvement of relatives:**
   - Palliative care actively involves relatives in the care process. Training and resources are provided to facilitate at-home care if that is the patient's desire.

9. **Grief counselling:**
   - After the patient's death, palliative care often provides support and accompaniment to the family during the grieving process.

Palliative care can be provided at any stage of a serious illness and is not limited to the last stage of life. It focuses on ensuring the best possible quality of life for patients and their families, regardless of the prognosis of the disease.

Parent Counseling

Parent counseling is an important part of many professional practices, including occupational therapy. Here are some features of parent counseling in the context of occupational therapy:

1. **Information exchange:**
    - Occupational therapists can educate parents about the therapy process, including goals, methods, and expected progress.
    - Information about the child's specific needs and challenges can also be shared.
2. **Family Resources and Strengthening:**
    - Parent counseling in occupational therapy often involves the identification and use of family resources. This may include strengthening family support systems.
    - Parents are encouraged to recognize and strengthen their role as their child's primary supporter.
3. **Development Promotion:**
    - Occupational therapists can help parents deepen their understanding of their child's normal development.
    - Counseling can focus on how parents can support their child's development through activity-based approaches in everyday life.
4. **Parent-Child Interaction:**
    - Counseling may focus on fostering positive parent-child interactions to strengthen the relationship and support the implementation of therapeutic strategies in the home setting.
5. **Homework and exercises:**
    - Occupational therapists can recommend specific activities and exercises for parents to do at home to continue therapeutic goals outside of sessions.
    - Clear instructions and support in integrating therapeutic activities into everyday life are part of the counselling.

6. **Parenting skills:**
   - Counseling can focus on equipping parents with the necessary skills and strategies to manage their children's particular needs.
   - There can also be room for sharing parenting experiences and challenges.
7. **Collaboration and communication:**
   - Parent counseling often involves fostering open communication between parents and therapists.
   - Setting common goals and setting realistic expectations are important elements of cooperation.

So, parent counseling in occupational therapy is designed to create a supportive environment where parents are given the resources and knowledge to promote the best possible development and quality of life for their children.

Partial performance fault

The terms "partial performance disorder" or "partial performance deficit" are often used in the context of learning and developmental disorders to describe difficulties in specific cognitive areas. These difficulties can lead to certain tasks or activities being impaired in the school or work environment. These terms do not represent official medical diagnoses, but rather general descriptions of weaknesses in specific cognitive functions.

Here are some examples of partial performance failures:

1. **Dyslexia:** Difficulty reading, such as problems decoding words, difficulty understanding texts, or reversing letters.
2. **Dyscalculia:** Impairments in the mathematical field that may include difficulty understanding numbers, solving math problems, or learning mathematical concepts.
3. **Dysgraphia:** difficulties in writing, which can manifest themselves in illegible handwriting, problems with writing speed or difficulty structuring texts.
4. **Attention deficit/hyperactivity disorder (ADHD):** ADHD is often considered a partial performance disorder because it involves specific difficulties with attention, impulse control, and hyperactivity.
5. **Auditory processing disorder:** Difficulty processing and interpreting auditory information, which can lead to problems listening, understanding instructions, or distinguishing sounds.
6. **Visual perception disorder:** impairments in visual processing that can lead to difficulties in recognizing shapes, thinking spatially, or processing visual stimuli.

People with partial performance disorders are often very gifted and talented in other areas of their lives. Early identification and targeted interventions, such as special educational programs or therapeutic approaches, can help to overcome the challenges and promote individual strengths. A comprehensive approach that includes collaboration between parents, teachers, and professionals is often critical to providing support to children and adults with partial performance disorders.

Patient Counseling

Patient counseling is an essential part of healthcare and refers to communication between healthcare professionals and patients. The aim is to provide patients with comprehensive information, support and involvement in the decision-making process regarding their health care. Patient counseling includes:

1. **Communication:**
   - Effective communication is crucial. Medical staff should use clear, understandable language and ensure that patients understand the information.
2. **Information and education:**
   - Patients should be provided with comprehensive information about their health, diagnosis, planned treatments, risks and alternatives. Education enables patients to make informed decisions.
3. **Treatment Planning:**
   - In close cooperation with the patient, an individual treatment plan is created based on the specific needs, values and preferences.
4. **Questions:**
   - Patients often have questions and concerns about their health. Medical staff should be prepared to answer these questions and clarify any uncertainties.
5. **Empowerment:**
   - Patients should be encouraged to actively participate in their health care. This includes fostering self-management skills and encouraging information gathering.
6. **Emotional Support:**
   - Health challenges can be emotionally draining. Patient counselors also offer emotional support by addressing fears and concerns.
7. **Shared decision-making:**
   - Shared decision-making involves a collaborative approach, where patients and medical staff work

together to make decisions that meet individual needs.

8. **Cultural Sensitivity:**
   - Patient advisors should show cultural sensitivity and respect patients' cultural backgrounds to ensure effective communication.

9. **Documentation:**
   - Key information and conversations should be documented to ensure there is a comprehensive understanding of patient needs and continuity of care is ensured.

10. **Continuing education:**
    - Patient counseling may also include continuing education, where patients receive information about their disease, prevention, treatment options, and healthy lifestyle habits.

Patient counseling is a dynamic process that adapts to changing needs and advances in healthcare. Good patient counseling helps to increase patient satisfaction, improve treatment adherence, and ultimately achieve better health outcomes.

Pediatrics

Pediatrics is the medical specialty that focuses on the care of children and adolescents. The term "pediatrics" is derived from the Greek word "pais," which means "child," and "iatreia," which means "medicine" or "treatment." Pediatricians are physicians who specialize in caring for children and address the specific health needs of children and adolescents. Other information on pediatrics includes:

1. **Developmental Physiology:**
   - Pediatricians have a deep understanding of children's developmental physiology. This includes physical, emotional, cognitive, and social development from infancy to adolescence.
2. **Preventive medicine:**
   - One focus of pediatrics is preventive medicine. Pediatricians offer vaccinations, screenings, and advice on how to promote a healthy lifestyle.
3. **Growth and development:**
   - Pediatricians monitor children's growth and development to ensure they are developing normally and to detect any developmental disorders or delays early.
4. **Child Health Conditions:**
   - Pediatricians diagnose, treat, and care for children with various health conditions, ranging from infections to chronic conditions and genetic disorders.
5. **Acute illnesses and injuries:**
   - Pediatricians treat acute conditions such as respiratory infections, gastrointestinal disorders, and injuries that can occur in childhood.
6. **Neonatal care:**
   - Pediatrics also includes neonatal care, including monitoring preterm infants, caring for newborns in the intensive care unit, and advising parents on infant care.

7. **Adolescent Medicine:**
   - Pediatricians also specialize in adolescent health needs. This includes topics such as puberty, sexual health, mental health, and prevention of behavioral disorders.
8. **Vaccinations:**
   - Pediatricians play a critical role in administering immunization according to national immunization recommendations to protect children from infectious diseases.
9. **Advice for parents:**
   - Pediatricians provide parents with advice and guidance on topics such as nutrition, safety, sleep habits, behavior development, and other aspects of raising children.
10. **Multidisciplinary collaboration:**
    - Pediatricians often work with other professionals, including pediatric surgeons, pediatric cardiologists, child psychologists, and therapists, to ensure comprehensive care for children.

Pediatrics is a diverse specialty that deals with the care of children of different ages and health conditions. Working closely with parents and other healthcare professionals is an essential part of pediatric care to achieve the best possible outcomes for children's health and well-being.

PEO Model

The PEO model is a theoretical framework in occupational therapy that examines the interaction between three central aspects of human action: person, environment, and person-environment-occupation (PEO). This model helps occupational therapists understand the complex relationships between these three elements and analyze the impact on individuals' actions and participation.

1. **Person:** This aspect refers to the individual seeking occupational therapy interventions. The person includes physical, psychological, social, and spiritual characteristics. These can be skills, limitations, interests, values, and preferences that influence a person's actions.
2. **Environment:** The environment represents the context in which the person operates. This includes both physical and social aspects. These include housing conditions, workplace, social relationships, cultural factors and social structures. The environment can be conducive or hindering a person's ability to act.
3. **Occupation:** This refers to the actions or activities that a person performs to complete their daily tasks. This can range from everyday activities such as dressing, eating, and working, to leisure activities and social interactions.

The PEO model emphasizes the interactions between these three elements. It argues that a person's actions depend not only on their individual characteristics, but also on the way in which the environment is designed and what the requirements of the tasks are.

Occupational therapists use the PEO model to conduct comprehensive assessments that take into account all three elements and to develop interventional approaches aimed at improving a person's agency capacity in their particular context. Through this holistic approach, the PEO model helps to better understand individual needs and develop appropriate, client-centered interventions.

Perception

In occupational therapy, perception plays a central role, as it forms the basis for the performance of various activities in daily life. Perception refers to the ability to absorb, interpret and organize information from the environment and one's own body. It encompasses various aspects, including sensory perception, cognitive perception, and social perception.

1. **Sensory perception:** This aspect refers to the processing of sensory inputs such as sight, hearing, touch, taste, and smell. In occupational therapy, techniques are used to promote sensory integration, that is, the effective processing of sensory impressions to enable appropriate responses and behaviors.
2. **Cognitive perception:** This is the processing of information at higher cognitive levels, including attention, memory, problem-solving, and judgment. In occupational therapy, cognitive strategies and exercises are used to improve cognitive abilities and promote independence in everyday activities.
3. **Social cognition:** This aspect refers to how people interpret social information, such as the ability to understand nonverbal cues, recognize social norms, and maintain relationships. In occupational therapy, social skills can be trained to improve social integration and interaction.

Nurturing perception is crucial to help people optimize their abilities and live as independent and fulfilling a life as possible. Occupational therapists use targeted exercises, activities, and strategies that are tailored to the individual needs and goals of their clients.

Perception enhancement

Perceptual enhancement refers to actions and interventions aimed at improving a person's ability to perceive and interpret sensory impressions. These interventions can be applied in various therapeutic areas, including occupational therapy. Points of perception promotion:

1. **Sensory Integration:**
    - Sensory integration is a therapeutic approach that aims to organize and process sensory stimuli. Through targeted exercises and activities, sensory experiences are used to improve perceptual skills.
2. **Visual Perception Enhancement:**
    - Measures to improve visual perception focus on the ability to interpret visual stimuli. This can include activities such as recognizing shapes, colors, sizes, and spatial relationships.
3. **Auditory Perception Enhancement:**
    - Here, the focus is on improving auditory processing and interpretation of sounds. Exercises may include distinguishing sounds, locating sounds, and processing spoken information.
4. **Tactile Perception Enhancement:**
    - Tactile perception enhancement focuses on the senses of touch. This can include improving the ability to distinguish textures, temperatures, and pressure.
5. **Proprioceptive Perception Promotion:**
    - Proprioceptive perception refers to the ability to perceive the position and movement of one's own body in space. Exercises can improve sensitivity to muscle tension and joint movements.
6. **Promoting balance and vestibular perception:**
    - These measures aim to improve balance and spatial orientation. Exercises may include training the vestibular system (organ of balance in the inner ear) and stabilizing balance.

7. **Integration of multiple senses:**
    - Comprehensive interventions can aim to integrate multiple senses at the same time in order to achieve comprehensive perceptual promotion. This can be especially important when it comes to complex tasks or activities of daily living.
8. **Everyday activities:**
    - The integration of perceptual exercises into everyday activities makes it possible to apply the acquired skills in practical situations.

The selection of specific perception enhancement measures depends on a person's individual needs and challenges. Occupational therapists and other professionals can develop targeted interventions to strengthen perceptual skills and improve quality of life.

Phonological awareness

Phonological awareness refers to the ability to recognize, understand, and manipulate the sounds in spoken language. This ability is crucial for acquiring reading and writing. Phonological awareness encompasses various aspects, including:

1. **Phonemic identification:** The ability to identify sounds (phonemes) in spoken language. This may include hearing, distinguishing, and recognizing sounds as they occur in words.
2. **Phonemic segmentation:** The ability to divide words into individual sounds or syllables. For example, the ability to divide the word "cat" into the sounds /k/, /a/ and /t/.
3. **Phonemic manipulation:** The ability to manipulate sounds in a word by adding, removing, or replacing them. This can be done, for example, by adding a sound to "house" to "mouse".
4. **Rhymes:** The ability to identify words that have similar sounding endings. For example, recognizing that "hat" and "cap" rhyme.
5. **Hyphenation:** The ability to divide words into syllables. This is important because syllables affect the rhythmic and phonological flow of words.

Phonological awareness is a crucial precursor to the acquisition of reading skills. Children who have good phonological awareness often have an easier start learning to read. Difficulties with phonological awareness may indicate reading and writing difficulties.

Phonological awareness can be developed through targeted exercises and activities. In the school environment, phonological awareness programs are often used to provide children with a solid foundation for reading and writing.

Physiotherapy

Physiotherapy, also known as physical therapy or physical therapy, is a form of therapeutic intervention aimed at improving the body's ability to move and function, relieve pain and promote quality of life. This form of therapy is used for a variety of health problems, whether due to injuries, orthopedic diseases, neurological disorders or other health conditions. Here are some features of physiotherapy:

1. **Micromotion study:**
    - Physiotherapists perform a detailed analysis of the patient's motor functions to identify possible limitations, dysfunctions or sources of pain.
2. **Individual therapy plan:**
    - Based on the movement analysis, physiotherapists develop an individual therapy plan that is tailored to the specific needs and goals of the patient.
3. **Exercises and rehabilitation:**
    - Physiotherapy involves targeted exercises to strengthen muscles, improve joint mobility and promote coordination. This can include both active and passive exercises.
4. **Manual therapy:**
    - Manual techniques, such as mobilization or massage, are used to treat joint and soft tissue problems and promote blood circulation.
5. **Posture improvement:**
    - Physiotherapists often work on correcting postural problems in order to optimize the load on joints and muscles.
6. **Respiratory therapy:**
    - In certain cases, especially in the case of respiratory problems or after surgery, respiratory therapy can be part of physiotherapy.
7. **Pain management:**
    - Physical therapy may include pain management techniques to reduce pain and improve quality of life.

8. **Neurological rehabilitation:**
    - In the case of neurological disorders, such as strokes or neurological injuries, physiotherapy can help improve motor skills and independence.
9. **Gait analysis:**
    - Gait analysis can be part of physical therapy, especially for orthopedic or neurological problems, to identify and treat gait disorders.
10. **Counselling and patient education:**
    - Physiotherapists often offer advice and education about the specific diagnosis, treatment plan and preventive measures.

Physiotherapy is performed by specially trained physiotherapists and can take place in a variety of settings, including hospitals, rehabilitation centres, doctors' offices or even in the home environment. It is an integrative component in rehabilitation after injuries or operations and plays a key role in the treatment of chronic diseases.

Pressure ulcer prophylaxis

Pressure ulcer prophylaxis refers to measures and strategies to prevent pressure ulcers, also known as pressure ulcers or bedsores. Pressure ulcers occur when tissue is damaged due to prolonged pressure, friction, or moisture, especially in areas with little subcutaneous fatty tissue over bone prominences such as the hips, heels, elbows, and sacrum.

Here are some key approaches to pressure ulcer prophylaxis:

1. **Regular repositioning:** People who are bedridden or in wheelchairs should be repositioned regularly to relieve pressure on certain areas of the body. The frequency of relocation depends on the individual risk and condition.
2. **Optimal positioning:** Proper positioning and positioning of the body are crucial to minimize pressure points. Special positioning aids such as cushions and foam pads can be used.
3. **Skin care:** The skin should be checked regularly for signs of redness, swelling, or changes. Good skin care, including cleansing and moisturizing, is important to keep the skin intact.
4. **Suitable mattresses and seat cushions:** The use of special mattresses and seat cushions with pressure relief properties can help reduce the risk of pressure ulcers.
5. **Nutrition:** A balanced diet with adequate hydration is important to support skin health and promote wound healing.
6. **Promoting physical activity:** Promoting movement and mobility as much as possible helps to reduce pressure on certain areas of the body.
7. **Training of nursing staff:** Nursing staff in hospitals, care facilities and home care should be trained in pressure ulcer prophylaxis in order to implement appropriate measures.
8. **Pressure distribution materials:** Using special materials such as anti-decubitus mattresses or seat cushions can help reduce pressure on vulnerable areas of the skin.

Pressure ulcer prophylaxis is especially important in people with limited mobility, chronic conditions, the elderly, and others who are at increased risk of pressure ulcers. Individual risk factors and needs should be taken into account when developing prevention strategies. When caring for people at high risk of pressure ulcers, close cooperation between patients, relatives and caregivers is of great importance.

Preventative care

Preventative care is a benefit provided by long-term care insurance in Germany that serves to temporarily relieve the burden on family caregivers. It allows a substitute caregiver to step in for the caregiver if the caregiver is temporarily prevented from taking over the care and support. Preventative care is intended to help family caregivers take necessary time off, for example for vacation, recreation or illness.

Some important points regarding preventative care:

1. **Duration of the benefit:** Preventative care can be used for a maximum of 42 days per calendar year. If the full service was not used in the previous year, the rest can be used in the current year.
2. **Financing:** The costs for preventative care are covered by long-term care insurance. A certain budget is available for this purpose, which is based on the level of care of the person to be cared for.
3. **Type of service:** Preventative care can be provided in the form of hourly support by an outpatient care service or by a substitute caregiver who temporarily takes over the care.
4. **Eligibility requirements:** In order to be entitled to preventative care, the person to be cared for must have a degree of care. The caregiver must be prevented by the care in such a way that he or she is temporarily unable to provide care or can only provide it partially.
5. **Application:** The use of preventative care requires a prior application to the long-term care insurance fund. This should be done in advance in order to be able to organize the services in time.

Preventative care is an important support for family caregivers in order to maintain their own health and maintain the care situation in the long term. It is advisable to find out about the possibilities and conditions of preventative care at an early stage and, if necessary, to take the appropriate steps.

Proprioceptive Neuromuscular Facilitation (PNF)

PNF stands for "Proprioceptive Neuromuscular Facilitation" and is a therapeutic approach based on improving movement and functional abilities. The PNF method was developed by physiotherapists Herman Kabat, Irmgard Bartenieff and Margaret Knott. The focus is on promoting movement by stimulating the neuromuscular system. Other features of the PNF:

1. **Proprioception:**
   - Proprioception refers to the perception of one's body's position and movement in space. PNF uses proprioceptive stimuli to improve movement control.
2. **Neuromuscular Activation:**
   - PNF focuses on improving the interaction between muscles and the nervous system. Certain movement patterns trigger reflexive reactions that promote muscle activity.
3. **Diagonal Pattern:**
   - A characteristic feature of the PNF is the diagonal movement patterns. These patterns mimic natural movements of daily life and are designed to activate multiple muscle groups at once.
4. **Stimulation of motor skills:**
   - PNF uses various techniques to stimulate motor control. These include, but are not limited to, stretching techniques, resistance exercises, and diagonal movement patterns.
5. **Accentuated movement patterns:**
   - PNF emphasizes emphasized movement patterns, where the patient performs specific movements while the therapist provides resistance or support.
6. **Promoting Stability:**
   - By activating muscle groups in a coordinated manner, the stability of the body is improved. This can be especially beneficial for people with neurological conditions or injuries.

7. **Improving flexibility:**
   - PNF also includes techniques to improve flexibility by incorporating muscle stretches and passive movements.
8. **Patient involvement:**
   - Patients are actively involved in the therapy process. You will be guided to perform certain movement patterns in order to achieve the desired neuromuscular responses.
9. **Applicability in various areas:**
   - PNF is used in rehabilitation after injuries, for neurological diseases such as stroke or for orthopaedic problems. It is also used in sports physiotherapy to improve performance.
10. **Individualization of therapy:**
    - PNF therapy is often individually tailored to the patient's needs. Therapists tailor techniques according to specific constraints and goals.

The PNF method has been shown to be effective in improving movement, muscle control, and functional abilities. It is used by physiotherapists, occupational therapists and other professionals in rehabilitation to optimize the motor function and quality of life of their patients.

Psychiatry

Psychiatry is a medical specialty that deals with the diagnosis, treatment, and prevention of mental illness. Psychiatrists are doctors who specialize in psychiatry and focus on the study, diagnosis, and treatment of mental disorders. Psychiatry includes, among other things:

1. **Mental disorders:**
    - Psychiatry deals with a variety of mental disorders, including anxiety disorders, mood disorders (such as depression and bipolar disorder), schizophrenia, eating disorders, personality disorders, and many others.
2. **Diagnostics:**
    - Psychiatrists use clinical interviews, standardized questionnaires, and other diagnostic tools to diagnose mental disorders. Diagnosis is based on the symptoms reported by patients, as well as observations and evaluations by the doctor.
3. **Therapeutic approaches:**
    - Therapy in psychiatry can include a variety of approaches, including drug therapy (psychotropic drugs), psychotherapy, electroconvulsive therapy (ECT), and other somatic therapies. The selection of the appropriate approach depends on the type of disorder and the individual needs of the patient.
4. **Psychotherapy:**
    - Psychiatrists can use psychotherapeutic techniques to help patients cope with emotional difficulties, interpersonal problems, and changes in behavior. Various forms of psychotherapy, such as cognitive behavioral therapy or psychodynamic therapy, are used.
5. **Drug treatment:**
    - The prescription of psychotropic drugs is a common practice in psychiatry. Medication can help relieve symptoms and stabilize emotional balance.

6. **Disease prevention:**
    - Psychiatrists can also take preventive measures to reduce the risk of mental illness. This may include information campaigns, early detection and intervention for risk factors.
7. **Interdisciplinary cooperation:**
    - Psychiatrists often work with other healthcare professionals, including psychologists, social workers, nurse practitioners, and therapists, to provide comprehensive care for patients with mental health disorders.
8. **Research:**
    - Psychiatrists participate in research activities to deepen the understanding of mental disorders, develop new therapeutic approaches, and improve the effectiveness of treatments.
9. **Crisis intervention:**
    - Psychiatrists can intervene in emergencies and manage acute crisis situations. This may include assessment of suicidality, acute psychotic episodes, or other emergency situations.

Psychiatry plays an important role in promoting mental health and improving the quality of life of people with mental illness. A multidisciplinary approach, which includes different therapeutic modalities, is often used to meet the individual needs of patients.

Psychoeducation

Psychoeducation refers to an educational approach that aims to educate individuals and their families about mental health, mental disorders, and therapeutic interventions. The purpose of psychoeducation is to provide knowledge to promote understanding, acceptance, and management of mental health issues. Here are some points of psychoeducation:

1. **Information transfer:**
    - Psychoeducation provides information about various aspects of mental health, including normal emotional functioning, symptoms of mental disorders, causes, progression, and treatment options.
2. **Reduction of stigma:**
    - By providing knowledge about mental health, psychoeducation can help reduce stigma and prejudice. By helping people better understand that mental health problems are just as real and treatable as physical illnesses, the stigma can be reduced.
3. **Promoting self-management:**
    - Psychoeducation empowers individuals to better manage their own mental health. This may include identifying stressors, developing coping strategies, and promoting a healthy lifestyle.
4. **Family involvement:**
    - In many cases, psychoeducation also involves family members and other supportive individuals. This promotes understanding and support for people with mental health issues.
5. **Early detection and prevention:**
    - By teaching warning signs and early detection criteria, people can learn to recognize signs of mental disorders in themselves or others. This allows for early intervention and prevention.
6. **Improvement of therapy adherence:**
    - When people have a better understanding of their mental health issues and the underlying treatment

options, they are more likely to actively participate in their therapy and take the recommended actions.

7. **Application for various disorders:**
   - Psychoeducation can be used for a variety of mental disorders, including depression, anxiety disorders, bipolar disorder, schizophrenia, and eating disorders.

8. **Group and individual settings:**
   - Psychoeducation can be carried out in both group and individual settings. Group sessions provide an opportunity to share experiences and support each other.

9. **Resource Brokerage:**
   - In addition to pure knowledge transfer, resources and support services can also be presented in psychoeducation sessions to facilitate access to further support services for those affected.

10. **Adaptation to individual needs:**
    - Psychoeducation can be adapted to the individual needs and requirements of the target group. This may include cultural, age-specific, or linguistic adjustments.

Psychoeducation is an integral part of the holistic treatment of mental health problems.

Psychomotor skills

Psychomotor skills refers to the interaction between psychological (mental) and motor (physical) activity. The term encompasses the integration of cognitive, emotional, and motor aspects into an individual's behavior. Psychomotor skills play an important role in human development and affect various areas, including physical and mental health. Here are some characteristics of psychomotricity:

1. **Motor development:**
   - Psychomotor skills are closely related to motor development, which includes advances in gross and fine motor skills, as well as coordination of movements. This is especially important in the early years of life, when children acquire basic motor skills.
2. **Cognitive and Emotional Aspects:**
   - Psychomotor skills integrate cognitive (mental) and emotional (emotional) aspects with motor skills. For example, solving a problem (cognitive) can be combined with a physical action (motor).
3. **Sensory Integration:**
   - Psychomotor skills include the ability to integrate and respond to sensory information from the environment. This can include processing visual, auditory, tactile, and kinesthetic stimuli.
4. **Movement as expression:**
   - Movement can serve as an expression of emotions. Psychomotor activity, for example, can help reduce stress or relieve emotional tension.
5. **Learning:**
   - Psychomotor skills play a role in learning processes. Through actions and movements, people can explore their surroundings, acquire new skills, and gain experiences.
6. **Therapeutic Applications:**
   - In therapy, especially in areas such as occupational therapy and psychomotor therapy, psychomotor skills are used to promote development, improve

motor skills, and address emotional or cognitive challenges.

7. **Professional Application:**
   - In some professional contexts, such as sports, art or music, psychomotor skills play an important role in optimizing performance and expressiveness.

8. **Influence on social behavior:**
   - Psychomotor skills can influence social behavior. The ability to move and express oneself appropriately can play a role in social interactions.

9. **Age and development:**
   - The importance of psychomotor skills varies according to age and stage of development. In childhood, the focus is on the acquisition of basic motor skills, while in adulthood, the integration of movement and cognitive processes plays a role.

10. **Holistic approach:**
    - Psychomotor skills are often considered part of a holistic approach to promoting health and well-being. This includes physical, emotional, and cognitive aspects.

In various therapeutic, pedagogical and professional disciplines, psychomotor skills are used to support the development and well-being of people. The integration of psychic and motor skills is a complex process that affects different dimensions of human existence.

Quality management

Quality management refers to the systematic process by which organizations ensure that their products or services meet or exceed the set quality standards. The goal of quality management is to ensure customer satisfaction, improve the efficiency and effectiveness of processes, and promote continuous improvement within the organization. Further information from Quality Management:

1. **Quality Standards & Goals:**
   - Organizations set quality standards that define the minimum requirements for their products or services. Quality objectives are formulated to ensure that these standards are met or exceeded.
2. **Quality Management System (QMS):**
   - A QMS is a structured system of policies, processes, and procedures designed to manage quality in all areas of an organization. It ensures that the quality objectives are systematically pursued and achieved.
3. **Customer orientation:**
   - Customer orientation is a central aspect of quality management. Organizations should understand what quality requirements their customers have and align their products or services accordingly.
4. **Process orientation:**
   - Quality management places a strong focus on the processes within an organization. Efficient and effective processes help to ensure quality and use resources efficiently.
5. **Risk management:**
   - Identifying, assessing and managing risks are important aspects of quality management. This includes analysing risks that could affect quality and taking steps to minimise them.
6. **Measurement and monitoring:**
   - Quality management involves the regular measurement and monitoring of processes and results to ensure that quality standards are met. This

is often done through the use of performance indicators and quality measurements.

7. **Continuous Improvement:**
   - The principle of continuous improvement is crucial in quality management. Organizations strive to constantly improve their processes and products based on feedback, experience, and new insights.

8. **Training & Development:**
   - Training and development of employees are important elements of quality management. Well-trained employees understand the organization's quality goals and can help achieve them.

9. **Documentation and Records:**
   - Clear documentation of processes, procedures and results is crucial in quality management. This facilitates traceability, traceability and verifiability of quality aspects.

10. **Certification:**
    - In some industries, certification according to international quality standards, such as ISO 9001, is an important step in quality management. These certifications show that an organization meets certain quality requirements.

Implementing effective quality management helps to increase competitiveness, increase customer trust, and ensure the long-term stability of an organization.

Quality of life

Quality of life refers to a person's overall well-being in various areas of life. It is a comprehensive concept that takes into account not only physical health, but also social, emotional, mental, economic and environmental factors. Quality of life is subjective and can be perceived differently from person to person. Here are some of the key factors that can affect quality of life:

1. **Bless you:**
   - Physical health plays a central role in quality of life. This includes aspects such as physical fitness, freedom from disease, adequate sleep and nutrition.
2. **Psychological well-being:**
   - Emotional and mental well-being is an important factor. This includes feelings of happiness, contentment, stress management, and the ability to cope with challenges.
3. **Social Relationships:**
   - The quality of interpersonal relationships contributes significantly to the quality of life. Strong social support, family relationships, friendships, and community integration all play a role.
4. **Job satisfaction:**
   - Satisfaction with one's professional activity and work situation has a significant impact on the quality of life.
5. **Financial stability:**
   - Economic factors, such as financial security, income and access to resources, can affect quality of life.
6. **Education:**
   - Access to education and the opportunity for personal development have an impact on the quality of life.
7. **Leisure and recreation:**
   - The ability to have time for recreation and leisure activities contributes to the quality of life.

8. **Environmental quality:**
    - The environment in which one lives, including air and water quality, safety, and access to green spaces, can affect the quality of life.
9. **Cultural and spiritual factors:**
    - Cultural and spiritual beliefs and practices can contribute to personal well-being and quality of life.
10. **Autonomy and self-determination:**
    - The ability to self-determine and the feeling of control over one's own life have a positive influence on the quality of life.

Quality of life is often measured through subjective assessments and self-reports by the people concerned. However, there are also standardized tools and surveys that are used to measure quality of life in different contexts. An improved quality of life is often formulated as a goal in various areas of health care, social services, and policy.

It is significant that quality of life is a multidimensional concept and individual priorities and values should be taken into account. What is considered a high quality of life for one person may be different for another.

Reconstructive Therapy

Restorative therapy in occupational therapy refers to a therapeutic approach that aims to restore or improve the functional abilities and skills of people who are impaired due to illness, injury, or other health impairments. The main goal of restorative therapy is to optimize the individual functional status and promote independence in everyday activities.

This form of therapy focuses on rehabilitation and building specific skills that have been lost or impaired due to physical, cognitive, or psychological challenges. Various methods and techniques are used to promote motor skills, cognitive function, sensory integration and other relevant areas.

Reconstructive therapy in occupational therapy takes into account the individual needs and goals of the patient and is carried out in close cooperation with the therapist. The doctor develops a tailor-made therapy plan that is tailored to the specific impairments and goals of the individual. Through targeted exercises, activities and interventions, the aim is to achieve the recovery of lost or impaired abilities in order to support the patient in leading a life that is as independent and fulfilled as possible.

Regulatory disorder

Regulatory disorder refers to difficulties in regulating emotions, behavior, and sensory stimuli. These difficulties can occur in children and are often referred to as regulatory disorder of the sensory processing and regulatory area or as a disorder of emotional self-regulation.

Some aspects that may be associated with regulatory disorders:

1. **Emotional dysregulation: Difficulty** recognizing, expressing, and regulating emotions. Children with regulatory disorders may have excessive outbursts of anger, mood swings, or difficulty calming down.
2. **Behavioral problems:** Challenges in controlling impulsive behavior or difficulty adapting to social norms. This can lead to problems in social interactions, at school, or in the home environment.
3. **Sensory processing difficulties:** hypersensitivity or undersensitivity to sensory stimuli such as sounds, touch, or visual sensations. This hypersensitivity or undersensitivity can lead to stressful situations.
4. **Problems with attention and concentration:** Difficulty maintaining attention and concentrating on certain tasks.
5. **Sleep and eating problems:** Regulatory disorders can also be associated with sleep problems, eating difficulties, or other basic functions of daily life.

Regulatory disorders are not limited to a particular behavior or emotion, but can encompass a wide range of challenges. These difficulties can affect the child's quality of life and affect various areas of life.

Intervention for regulatory disorders may require a multidisciplinary approach that includes psychological, educational, and sometimes occupational therapy or physiotherapy elements. Early identification and support are critical to encourage the development of healthy coping strategies and minimize long-term impacts. Parents, teachers, and professionals can work together to develop individualized support plans.

Rehab Management

Rehab management refers to the coordinated planning, organization, and monitoring of rehabilitation activities for people who need support due to illness, injury, or disability. The aim of rehabilitation management is to promote individual rehabilitation and ensure that affected individuals receive the best possible support to restore or improve their ability to function. Key aspects of rehab management:

1. **Needs assessment:**
   - The first step in rehab management is a comprehensive assessment of the individual's needs. This includes the assessment of the medical, psychological, social and professional aspects.
2. **Individual rehabilitation plan:**
   - Based on the needs assessment, an individual rehabilitation plan is drawn up. This plan sets out the goals, actions, and timeframes for rehabilitation and takes into account the specific needs and objectives of the individual.
3. **Interdisciplinary cooperation:**
   - Rehab management requires close collaboration between various professionals, including doctors, therapists, nurses, social workers, and others, to ensure comprehensive and coordinated care.
4. **Coordinated services:**
   - Rehab management coordinates various services, including medical care, therapy, nursing, social support, and vocational rehabilitation, to best meet the needs of the individual.
5. **Patient involvement:**
   - A central principle of rehabilitation management is the active participation of the patient in the rehabilitation process. This includes setting goals, adhering to therapy plans, and attending education and training.

6. **Continuous monitoring and adjustment:**
    - The rehabilitation process is continuously monitored and adjusted if necessary. This may include changes in rehabilitation goals, treatment plans, or support measures.
7. **Return to everyday life:**
    - Rehabilitation management aims to promote individual independence and participation in everyday life. Planning for a return to work or community can be an important part.
8. **Evaluation of the results:**
    - At the end of the rehabilitation process, an evaluation of the results achieved is carried out. This serves to check the success of the measures and, if necessary, to make adjustments for the future.
9. **Psychosocial support:**
    - Rehabilitation management also takes into account psychosocial aspects. This can include support for mental health challenges, involvement of family and social environment, and promotion of quality of life.
10. **Quality:**
    - The quality of the services provided within the framework of rehabilitation management is monitored and ensured. This includes adherence to standards, evaluation of patient satisfaction and continuous improvement of processes.

Rehab management is a comprehensive approach that can improve the quality of life of people facing health challenges. It emphasizes holistic care, individuality and the integration of different specialties in order to achieve optimal rehabilitation.

Rehabilitation

Rehabilitation is a comprehensive, multidisciplinary approach to supporting people whose health or functions are impaired due to illness, injury, or disability. The aim of rehabilitation is to promote individual independence, quality of life and participation in everyday life. Characteristics of rehabilitation:

1. **Holistic approach:**
    - Rehabilitation looks at the person as a whole and takes into account physical, psychological, social and professional aspects. It aims to address impairments in various areas of life.
2. **Individual needs:**
    - Each person has unique needs, and rehabilitation adapts to individual challenges and goals. The rehabilitation process is tailored to the specific needs and abilities of the affected person.
3. **Multidisciplinary collaboration:**
    - Rehabilitation involves the collaboration of various professionals, including doctors, therapists (physiotherapists, occupational therapists, speech therapists), nurses, psychologists, social workers and others, to ensure comprehensive care.
4. **Objectives and objectives:**
    - Clear, realistic and measurable goals are set as part of rehabilitation. These goals may include improving mobility, increasing independence, reducing pain, or restoring job skills.
5. **Stages of rehabilitation:**
    - Rehabilitation can be divided into different phases, including the acute phase (immediately after the illness or injury), the post-acute or subacute phase, and the long-term or chronic phase. Each phase requires different approaches and intervention strategies.

6. **Medical rehabilitation:**
    - This includes medical treatment and care to stabilize the state of health and promote recovery. Medical rehabilitation may include hospitalization, physical therapy, and medical interventions.
7. **Functional rehabilitation:**
    - Here, the focus is on restoring functions and capabilities. This often involves physical and occupational therapy approaches to improve mobility, coordination, and self-care skills.
8. **Social Rehabilitation:**
    - Social rehabilitation focuses on promoting social integration and participation in community life. This includes social activities, psychosocial support and integration into social networks.
9. **Vocational rehabilitation:**
    - The aim of vocational rehabilitation is to support people in returning to or remaining in working life. This may include training, reskilling, workplace adjustments, and career guidance.
10. **Long-term care and support:**
    - In some cases, rehabilitation requires long-term care and support to maintain the goals achieved and maintain quality of life.

Rehabilitation is a continuous process that aims to positively impact the lives of people facing health challenges.

Remotivational Therapy

Remotivation therapy is a form of psychosocial intervention that aims to motivate people to increase their enjoyment of life and quality of life. This form of therapy is often used for people who have lost their motivation and zest for life due to various life circumstances, illnesses or psychological challenges. Points of remotivation therapy are:

1. **Objective:**
   - The main goal of remotivational therapy is to help people rediscover their intrinsic motivation and experience positive changes in their lives. This can be done on different levels, including emotional, social, and cognitive aspects.
2. **Customization:**
   - The therapy is individually tailored to the needs and abilities of each person. The therapist takes into account the individual's personal circumstances, history, and specific challenges.
3. **Psychosocial support:**
   - Remotivational therapy provides psychosocial support to help people identify their own resources, broaden their perspectives, and find new ways of coping with problems.
4. **Self-esteem and self-efficacy:**
   - A central focus is on strengthening self-esteem and self-efficacy. Therapy aims to help people develop a positive self-image and restore confidence in their own abilities.
5. **Activation and participation:**
   - Remotivation therapy promotes activation and participation in positive activities. This can include artistic and creative expressions, as well as social activities that help regain joy and interest in life.
6. **Identification of interests:**
   - By identifying and promoting personal interests and hobbies, an attempt is made to arouse interest in meaningful activities that contribute to remotivation.

7. **Community and social inclusion:**
    - The therapy aims to promote social contacts and support integration into the community. This can be achieved through group activities, social gathering places and the development of supportive networks.
8. **Cognitive approaches:**
    - Cognitive approaches can be used to identify and change negative thought patterns. Therapy can help to strengthen positive mindsets and develop constructive perspectives.
9. **Evaluation and adaptation:**
    - The therapy process is continuously evaluated, and intervention strategies are adjusted as needed to ensure that therapy meets the person's needs.
10. **Sustainability:**
    - Remotivation therapy is not only aimed at short-term improvements, but also aims for long-term changes and a sustainable increase in quality of life.

Remotivation therapy can be applied in a variety of fields, including mental health, rehabilitation, elderly care, and other areas where promoting joie de vivre and motivation is important.

Resilience

Resilience refers to a person's ability to recover, adapt, and emerge stronger from stressful life situations, crises, or trauma. It is a dynamic trait that allows people to overcome challenges and thrive in the face of adversity. Some characteristics of resilience are:

1. **Resistance to stress:**
    - Resilient people are able to cope with stress and pressure without it affecting their long-term mental or physical health.
2. **Adaptability:**
    - Resilient individuals can flexibly adapt to different life circumstances and changes. They are able to develop new strategies to deal with life's challenges.
3. **Self-efficacy:**
    - Resilient individuals have a strong sense of self-efficacy. They believe that they can have an impact on their environment and their circumstances, and see difficulties as challenges that they can overcome.
4. **Optimism:**
    - An optimistic approach to life is a characteristic feature of resilient people. They tend to be positive about the future and hopeful, even in difficult times.
5. **Social support:**
    - The ability to seek and accept social support is an important part of resilience. Resilient people often have strong social networks that serve as a resource in times of need.
6. **Emotional Regulation:**
    - Resilient individuals are able to recognize, accept, and regulate their emotions. You can respond appropriately to stress without being overwhelmed by strong negative emotions.
7. **Acceptance of change:**
    - Resilience involves the ability to accept change, even if it is unforeseen or challenging. Adapting to new realities is an essential aspect.

8. **Solution orientation:**
   - Resilient people focus on finding solutions instead of focusing on problems. They are actively looking for ways to deal with difficulties.
9. **Self-reflection:**
   - The ability to self-reflect allows resilient people to learn from experience, understand their own reactions, and continuously evolve.
10. **Change of perspective:**
    - Resilient individuals can take a broader perspective and see opportunities for personal development and growth even in difficult times.

Resilience is not a static trait, but can be strengthened through various measures and strategies. Interventions aimed at fostering psychological resilience may include stress management training, social support, mindfulness practices, and therapeutic approaches.

Resource orientation

Resource orientation is an approach across disciplines that aims to draw attention and focus to existing resources and strengths, rather than focusing solely on deficits or problems. This approach is applied in various fields, including psychology, education, social work, and therapy. Characteristics of resource orientation:

1. **Strengths Focus:**
   - The central aspect of resource orientation is to focus on existing strengths and positive aspects. This allows for a positive perspective and promotes self-efficacy.
2. **Determination of resources:**
   - Resource orientation involves the active identification and determination of existing resources. These can be personal strengths, social support systems, skills, interests, and other positive aspects.
3. **Empowerment:**
   - By emphasizing resources, empowerment is encouraged. People are encouraged to recognize and use their own abilities to bring about positive change in their lives.
4. **Collaborative approach:**
   - Resource orientation fosters a collaborative approach between professionals and individuals seeking support. Together, existing resources are identified and strategies are developed to achieve goals.
5. **Promoting self-efficacy:**
   - By encouraging people to recognize and use their own resources, self-efficacy is strengthened. This helps individuals maintain confidence in their abilities and control over their own lives.
6. **Solution orientation:**
   - Resource orientation is often combined with a solution-oriented perspective. The focus is on finding positive solutions that build on existing resources, rather than focusing solely on problems.

7. **Cultural Sensitivity:**
   - Resource orientation takes into account cultural diversity and individuality. It acknowledges that resources can be different in different cultural contexts and individual life experiences.
8. **Preventive approach:**
   - Resource orientation can also include preventive aspects by helping to strengthen existing resources to proactively address potential challenges and problems.
9. **Strengthening social networks:**
   - The emphasis on resources often includes social networks as well. Strengthening social connections and relationships can be considered an important resource.
10. **Holistic approach:**
    - Resource orientation looks at people as a whole and takes into account physical, emotional, cognitive and social aspects. The holistic approach promotes a comprehensive view of the person.

Resource orientation is built into many therapeutic and pedagogical approaches and can help foster positive change by building on existing strengths.

Rheumatism

"Rheumatism" is a term used to describe a variety of diseases of the musculoskeletal system and connective tissue that are associated with pain, swelling and impaired function in joints, muscles, tendons and other structures. However, the term "rheumatism" is not specific and encompasses a wide range of rheumatic diseases.

Here are some of the most common forms of rheumatic diseases:

1. **Rheumatoid arthritis (RA):** An autoimmune disease in which the immune system mistakenly attacks the joints, causing inflammation, pain, swelling, and joint destruction.
2. **Osteoarthritis (OA):** Also known as degenerative joint disease, this condition occurs when the cartilage in the joints decreases over time, causing pain and restrictions on joint movement.
3. **Ankylosing spondylitis:** An inflammatory joint disease that mainly affects the spine and can lead to stiffness and pain.
4. **Gout:** Caused by a buildup of uric acid crystals in the joints, which can lead to sudden attacks of pain.
5. **Lupus (systemic lupus erythematosus):** An autoimmune disease that can affect various organs and tissues, including joints.
6. **Scleroderma:** A rare condition in which connective tissue hardens and affects the skin and internal organs.
7. **Ankylosing spondylitis:** An inflammatory joint disease that mainly affects the spine.

The symptoms of rheumatism can vary from person to person and depending on the type of rheumatic disease. The most common symptoms include pain, swelling, stiffness of the joints, limited mobility, and fatigue.

The diagnosis and treatment of rheumatism often requires the cooperation of various medical professionals such as rheumatologists, orthopedists, physiotherapists and pain management professionals. Treatment may include medication, physical therapy, lifestyle changes, and in some cases, surgery. Early diagnosis and adequate treatment can help alleviate symptoms and improve quality of life.

Rheumatoid arthritis

Rheumatoid arthritis (RA) is a chronic, inflammatory autoimmune disease that mainly affects the joints. In this condition, the immune system mistakenly attacks its own joints, leading to inflammation, pain, swelling, and ultimately joint damage. However, rheumatoid arthritis can also affect other organs and tissues in the body.

Here are some features and aspects of rheumatoid arthritis:

1. **Symptoms:** The most common symptoms include morning stiffness, pain, and swelling in the joints, especially in the hands and feet. Symptoms may develop gradually and worsen over time.
2. **Inflammation:** The inflammation in rheumatoid arthritis can lead to joint damage if not treated in time. Joints may swell, heat up, and be painful.
3. **Symmetry:** RA often affects joints on both sides of the body symmetrically. This means that if a joint on the left side is affected, the corresponding joint on the right side is likely to be affected as well.
4. **Systemic effects:** In addition to joints, RA can affect other organs, including the skin, eyes, lungs, heart, and blood vessels.
5. **Autoimmune disease:** Rheumatoid arthritis is an autoimmune disease in which the immune system mistakenly attacks the body's own tissues. The exact trigger for this immune system malfunction is not fully understood.
6. **Early detection and diagnosis:** Diagnosis is based on a combination of clinical signs, blood tests (such as rheumatoid factor and antibodies to citrullinated protein), and imaging tests such as X-rays.
7. **Treatment:** Treatment for rheumatoid arthritis aims to control inflammation, reduce pain, minimize joint damage, and improve quality of life. Drug therapy, physical therapy, lifestyle changes, and in some cases, surgery may be part of the treatment plan.

It is important to detect and treat rheumatoid arthritis early in order to minimize joint damage and improve the quality of life of those affected. Working with a rheumatologist and an interdisciplinary treatment team is critical to the long-term care of people with rheumatoid arthritis.

Self-control

Self-control in occupational therapy refers to an individual's ability to plan, organize, and control their own actions, decisions, and reactions. It is an important aspect of self-regulation and self-control that is developed and promoted in the context of occupational therapy. Self-control plays a central role in improving independence and coping with daily life.

Self-control in occupational therapy:

1. **Self-regulation:** This refers to the ability to recognize, understand, and control one's own emotions, behaviors, and reactions. Occupational therapy can teach techniques and strategies to strengthen self-regulation, especially in people with various psychological or neurological challenges.
2. **Self-organization:** Self-management also includes the ability to plan, organize, and structure tasks. This is crucial for the successful performance of everyday activities. People who have difficulties in this area can benefit from occupational therapy interventions to improve their organizational skills.
3. **Self-determination:** The ability to set one's own goals, make decisions and take responsibility for one's own actions is another aspect of self-control. Occupational therapists can help people strengthen their autonomy and regain control of their own lives.
4. **Feedback processing:** The ability to interpret feedback from the environment and respond to it appropriately is also part of self-control. This can be an important focus of occupational therapy work for people who have difficulties in perceiving or processing stimuli.

Promoting self-control through occupational therapy helps people to be better able to cope with their individual challenges and achieve a higher level of independence in their daily lives.

Self-management

Self-management refers to a person's ability to effectively manage and regulate their own behavior, emotions, and resources in order to achieve personal goals and deal with life's challenges. It involves consciously designing and organizing one's own life, setting goals, prioritizing tasks, developing self-motivation and taking responsibility for one's own well-being. Key aspects of self-management are:

1. **Objective:**
    - Self-management often starts with setting clear, achievable goals. Defining goals provides clear direction and motivation for action.
2. **Prioritization:**
    - The ability to prioritize tasks and differentiate between important and less important activities is critical to effective self-management.
3. **Time management:**
    - Effective time management is an important part of self-management. This includes planning activities, setting deadlines, and making efficient use of available time.
4. **Self-motivation:**
    - Self-management requires self-motivation. The ability to motivate yourself and keep going even in difficult times is critical to success.
5. **Homeostasis:**
    - Self-regulation refers to the ability to regulate emotions and behavior. This includes controlling stress, overcoming challenges, and promoting emotional stability.
6. **Self-confidence:**
    - Self-management requires self-confidence, i.e. the ability to understand oneself and one's strengths and weaknesses. This allows for realistic self-assessment and identification of areas for development.

7. **Decision-making:**
   - The ability to make decisions is an integral part of self-management. This includes weighing options, making informed decisions, and taking responsibility for the consequences.
8. **Flexibility:**
   - Self-management also requires flexibility. The ability to adapt to change and adapt to new circumstances is important in order to deal with different situations.
9. **Communication:**
   - Effective communication, both with yourself and with others, is crucial. This includes clearly articulating needs, being willing to ask for help, and understanding one's communication styles.
10. **Reflection:**
    - Self-management involves continuous reflection on one's own behavior, attitudes and goal achievement. This allows for continuous adaptation and further development.

Self-management is a lifelong skill that is relevant in various areas of life, including professional, personal, and health aspects. It is a dynamic process that requires continuous adaptation and improvement. People can strengthen their self-management skills through self-reflection, education, and the application of effective strategies.

Sensorimotor

"Sensorimotor" refers to the interaction between sensory perception and motor activity. Sensorimotor integration is a central concept in occupational therapy and other areas of health and developmental work.

Sensorimotor skills have two main components:

1. **Sensory (sensory):** This refers to the perception of sensory stimuli or information by the sensory organs. These include visual perception (seeing), auditory perception (hearing), gustatory perception (tasting), olfactory perception (smelling) and tactile perception (touching).
2. **Motor skills (motor):** This refers to the body's ability to respond to sensory stimuli with movements. It includes gross motor skills (such as walking or jumping) and fine motor skills (such as grasping or writing).

The integration of sensory stimuli and motor responses is crucial for the ability to navigate the environment, act effectively and respond appropriately to various stimulated situations. An effective interplay of sensory and motor skills allows people to explore their environment, perform tasks, and successfully manage social interactions.

In occupational therapy, sensorimotor integration is often specifically promoted, especially in children with developmental disorders or people with neurological impairments. Through targeted exercises and activities, an attempt is made to strengthen the perceptual abilities and bring them into line with the motor skills.

In general, the concept of sensorimotor skills plays an important role in various areas, including children's development, post-injury rehabilitation, treatment of people with sensory processing disorders, and support for people with neurological disorders.

Sensorimotor integration

Sensorimotor integration is a process in the brain that integrates information from the sensory organs and motor system to enable coordinated actions and responses. This process plays a crucial role in motor control, spatial orientation and interaction with the environment. Here are some key concepts of sensorimotor integration:

1. **Sensory receptors:**
   - Sensory receptors in the sensory organs (such as the eyes, ears, skin, and muscles) capture information about the environment and the body.
2. **Information processing:**
   - The brain processes this sensory information, interprets it and generates appropriate motor responses.
3. **Motor Control:**
   - Motor control refers to the nervous system's ability to control muscles and movements. Sensorimotor integration plays a key role in the coordination of these movements.
4. **Sense of balance (vestibular system):**
   - The vestibular system, located in the inner ear, is responsible for the perception of balance and movement. Sensorimotor integration takes into account information from this system.
5. **Proprioception:**
   - Proprioceptive receptors in muscles, tendons and joints provide information about the position and movement of the limbs. This is important for body awareness.
6. **Eye-Hand Coordination:**
   - Sensorimotor integration plays a role in eye-hand coordination, which is the ability to match visual information with motor actions.

7. **Tactile Perception:**
   - The perception of touch stimuli (tactile perception) is another aspect of sensorimotor integration. This includes the processing of pressure, vibration, temperature, and texture.
8. **Stages:**
   - Sensorimotor integration plays a central role during the different stages of development, especially in early childhood development. It influences the development of motor skills, hand-eye coordination and interaction with the environment.
9. **Fine motor skills and gross motor skills:**
   - It is also crucial for the development of fine motor skills (precise movements, e.g. dexterity) and gross motor skills (larger, physical movements, e.g. walking).
10. **Impairments and therapy:**
    - Problems with sensorimotor integration can lead to developmental delays, coordination problems, or difficulties in everyday activities. In such cases, sensorimotor integration therapy can be used to promote integration.

Sensorimotor integration is a complex process that forms the basis for effective interactions with the environment. In case of difficulties in this area, targeted therapy can help to improve sensorimotor integration and increase quality of life.

Sensorimotor skills

Sensorimotor function refers to the interaction between sensory perceptions and motor activities. This term encompasses the ability of the nervous system to receive information from the environment through the senses, process it and translate it into motor actions. Sensorimotor skills play a crucial role in the development of motor skills, coordination and interaction with the environment. Sensorimotor skills include:

1. **Sensory perception:**
   - Sensorimotor skills begin with the absorption of sensory information from the sensory organs. This includes seeing, hearing, feeling, smelling and tasting.
2. **Processing in the central nervous system:**
   - The sensory information received is processed in the central nervous system (brain and spinal cord). This is where the interpretation and integration of the sensory impressions takes place.
3. **Motor Response:**
   - Based on the processed sensory information, motor reactions are triggered. The nervous system controls the muscles and allows movements in response to the perceived sensory impressions.
4. **Balance and spatial orientation:**
   - Sensorimotor skills play a crucial role in the perception of balance and spatial orientation. The vestibular system in the inner ear is particularly important here.
5. **Hand-eye coordination:**
   - The ability to coordinate visual information with motor actions is called hand-eye coordination. This is a central aspect of sensorimotor skills.
6. **Proprioception:**
   - Proprioceptive receptors in muscles, tendons and joints provide information about the position and

movement of one's own body. This contributes to body awareness.
7. **Fine and gross motor skills:**
    - Sensorimotor skills influence the development of fine motor skills (precise movements, such as grasping small objects) and gross motor skills (larger, physical movements, such as walking or jumping).
8. **Stages:**
    - Sensorimotor skills play an important role during the various stages of development, especially in early childhood development. It affects the achievement of milestones such as turning, sitting, crawling, and walking.
9. **Control and coordination:**
    - Sensorimotor skills are crucial for controlling and coordinating movements. Effective sensorimotor skills enable precise and goal-oriented actions.
10. **Impairments and therapy:**
    - Sensorimotor problems can lead to developmental delays or difficulties in motor coordination. In such cases, sensorimotor therapy can be used to promote development.

Sensorimotor function is thus a complex interplay of sensory and motor processes that forms the basis for motor development and interaction with the environment. If necessary, targeted exercises and therapeutic approaches can be used to promote sensorimotor skills.

Sensory Integration Therapy

Sensory integration therapy (SIT) is a form of therapy that aims to treat sensory processing disorders in children and adults. Sensory processing disorders affect the ability of the nervous system to appropriately process and interpret information from the senses (sight, hearing, touch, taste, smell, and the sensation of body position and movement).

Points of Sensory Integration Therapy:

1. **Rationale:**
   - The basic principle of sensory integration therapy is that the ability to process sensory information forms the basis for everyday functions and activities.
2. **Sensory Integration:**
   - Sensory integration refers to the brain's ability to organize and interpret information from different sensory organs to guide meaningful responses and actions.
3. **Sensorimotor activities:**
   - Therapy involves sensorimotor activities aimed at stimulating the nervous system and promoting the integration of sensory information. These include movement, balance, and tactile activities.
4. **Customization:**
   - The therapy is individually tailored to the needs of each individual. The therapist observes the patient's behavior and responses to sensory stimuli in order to plan appropriate interventions.
5. **Promotion of perception and organization:**
   - The aim is to improve perceptual abilities and enable efficient organization of sensory information. This can help improve self-regulation and emotional balance.
6. **Consideration of all senses:**
   - Sensory integration therapy takes into account all the senses, including the vestibular sense (sense of balance and movement), the proprioceptive sense

(perception of body position) and the tactile sense (sensation of touch).

7. **Active participation:**
   - Patients are actively involved in the therapy process. This can include activities such as climbing, swinging, balancing, grasping, and other movement and sensory inputs.

8. **Focus on play:**
   - Especially with children, playful learning and exploration are often emphasized. Through games and activities, an attempt is made to promote sensory integration in a natural way.

9. **Coordinated cooperation:**
   - Sensory integration therapy requires close collaboration between therapists, patients and, if necessary, parents or caregivers to promote integration into everyday life.

10. **Applications in different conditions:**
    - The therapy is often used for children with developmental disabilities, attention deficit hyperactivity disorder (ADHD), autism spectrum disorders, learning disabilities, and other conditions.

The efficacy of sensory integration therapy continues to be debated in the scientific community. Still, many parents and therapists report positive outcomes, especially in children with certain sensory processing disorders. Individuals interested in this therapy should consult with qualified therapists and professionals.

Short

Short-term memory is a part of the human memory system that temporarily stores information and can access it quickly. It plays a crucial role in various cognitive processes, especially in the processing and retrieval of information in the immediate present. Compared to long-term memory, short-term memory is limited to a limited amount of information and a limited amount of time.

Here are some features and functions of short-term memory:

1. **Limited capacity:** Short-term memory can only store a limited number of items for a limited time. This capacity is usually about seven units (plus or minus two) according to the well-known Miller's law.
2. **Quick access:** Short-term memory allows quick access to the stored information, which is important for performing everyday tasks, such as reading a text or performing calculations.
3. **Active processing:** Information in short-term memory is actively processed, which means that it is not only passively stored, but also processed while it is conscious.
4. **Transient in nature:** Unlike long-term memory, which is used to store information for the long term, short-term memory is temporary. Information that is not processed or repeated can be quickly forgotten.
5. **Working memory:** The term "working memory" is often used interchangeably with short-term memory. It refers to the ability to hold information while performing mental processes such as thinking, problem-solving, or decision-making.

Short-term memory is integral to many everyday cognitive tasks, from simple activities to complex mental performances. It also plays an important role in the learning process, as information usually passes through short-term memory before potentially transitioning into long-term memory.

Sigmatism

Sigmatism refers to a speech disorder in which the phoneme "S" (sigma) is not pronounced correctly. This disorder affects the articulation of the letter "S", as well as sometimes similar sounds such as "Z" or "Sch". Sigmatism is often referred to as a lisp.

There are several types of sigmatism, including:

1. **Interdental sigmatism:**
   - In this form, articulation occurs in which the tip of the tongue looks through between the incisors. This causes the sound of the letter "S" to be distorted or altered.
2. **Lateral sigmatism:**
   - Here, the sound of the letter "S" is influenced by a lateral position of the tongue, creating a lisping sound.
3. **Palatal Sigmatism:**
   - In this form, the tip of the tongue touches the hard palate, resulting in an inaccurate pronunciation of the sound "S".

Sigmatism often occurs in children during language development, but it can also occur in adults. In many cases, sigmatism disappears over time, especially as children grow older and improve their articulation skills. However, if the sigmatism persists for a long period of time and affects speech intelligibility, it may be useful to seek professional help from a speech therapist or speech therapist.

Therapy for sigmatism can include various exercises and techniques aimed at training the correct tongue position and articulation of the sound "S". The exact approach depends on the specific form of sigmatism and the individual needs of the person concerned.

Social integration

Social integration refers to the process by which people are integrated into a community or society. This integration involves participation in social, economic, cultural and political activities within the community. The term encompasses various aspects of social inclusion and the involvement of individuals in the fabric of society. Further information on social integration:

1. **Participation in community life:**
   - Social inclusion means active participation in various aspects of community life, including social events, activities, cultural events, and social interactions.
2. **Access to resources:**
   - It includes access to basic resources such as education, health care, employment opportunities, and social services to enable full and active participation in social life.
3. **Equality and inclusion:**
   - Social integration strives for equality and inclusion by ensuring that all members of society have the same rights, opportunities, and access, regardless of gender, ethnicity, social background, or other characteristics.
4. **Community identity:**
   - Developing a community identity, in which people experience a sense of belonging and connectedness to their community, is an essential part of social integration.
5. **Exchange of values and norms:**
   - Social integration involves the exchange of values, norms and cultural practices within society. This fosters a common understanding and cohesion.
6. **Social Networks and Relationships:**
   - The formation of social networks and relationships is crucial for social integration. This includes family relationships, friendships, professional contacts, and other social connections.

7. **Participation in the labour market:**
    - Integration into the labour market is an important aspect of social integration. This includes opportunities for employment, career advancement and economic contribution to society.
8. **Social acceptance:**
    - Social integration also includes social acceptance and respect for diversity. This includes acknowledging and appreciating different lifestyles, beliefs, and backgrounds.
9. **Social mobility:**
    - The possibility of social mobility, where individuals can improve their social position over time, is a goal of social integration.
10. **Citizen participation:**
    - The willingness and ability to participate in political processes and civil rights is another important aspect of social integration.

Promoting social inclusion is crucial for a just, inclusive and harmonious society. It is a continuous process that requires collaboration on an individual, community and societal level.

Social reintegration

Social reintegration refers to the process of reintegrating individuals into society who were previously excluded, isolated, or marginalized for various reasons. This process is often associated with people returning from the penitentiary system, health care, rehabilitation, the military, or other areas of life where they were temporarily disconnected from society. Here are some key aspects of social reintegration:

1. **Goal:**
    - The main goal of social reintegration is to reintegrate people who have been excluded from society for various reasons into the social fabric. This can happen after prison sentences, hospitalizations, military service, or other life events.
2. **Support System:**
    - An effective social reintegration process requires a supportive network that takes into account individual needs and challenges. These may include family support, community programs, psychosocial care, and vocational rehabilitation.
3. **Education & Training:**
    - Providing education and training opportunities is crucial to improve the skills and qualifications of those affected. This can increase their chances of professional success and social integration.
4. **Vocational rehabilitation:**
    - The promotion of vocational skills and the provision of vocational rehabilitation play an important role in social reintegration. This includes job search assistance, training, and creating professional opportunities.
5. **Psychosocial support:**
    - Psychosocial support plays a central role in social reintegration. Individuals may need support in coping with emotional and social challenges in order to successfully return to the community.

6. **Apartment and accommodation:**
   - Providing safe and stable housing is important to lay the foundation for successful social reintegration.
7. **Health care:**
   - Access to health care, including mental health services, is critical to addressing individual needs and promoting health and well-being.
8. **Community participation:**
   - The promotion of community participation and social engagement supports social inclusion. This can be done through volunteering, membership in social groups, or involvement in local activities.
9. **Life Skills Development:**
   - The promotion of life skills such as communication, conflict resolution and decision-making contributes to successful social reintegration.
10. **Legal support:**
    - In some cases, legal support may be necessary to ensure that individual rights are protected and legal barriers to social reintegration are overcome.

Social reintegration is a complex process that requires individualized support. A holistic approach that includes education, vocational rehabilitation, psychosocial support, and community integration is critical to achieving long-term positive outcomes.

Social Skills

Social competence refers to a person's ability to interact effectively with others and act successfully in social situations. It encompasses a set of skills that allow a person to build and maintain relationships and make positive social connections. Characteristics of social competence:

1. **Empathy:**
    - Empathy is the ability to empathize with other people's feelings and perspectives. It enables understanding of the emotions of others and fosters empathetic interpersonal relationships.
2. **Communication skills:**
    - Effective communication is crucial for social skills. These include listening, the ability to send clear messages, verbal and non-verbal communication, and the ability to express oneself clearly.
3. **Ability to cooperate:**
    - The ability to collaborate and work in a team is an important aspect of social skills. This includes a willingness to collaborate with others, resolve conflicts, and achieve common goals.
4. **Homeostasis:**
    - Self-regulation refers to the ability to recognize, understand, and control one's emotions. This allows for an appropriate response in various social situations.
5. **Intercultural Competence:**
    - In a globalized world, the ability to deal with people from different cultural backgrounds is of great importance. This requires intercultural sensitivity and adaptability.
6. **Social Intelligence:**
    - Social intelligence includes understanding social situations, reading social signals, and adapting behavior to different social contexts.

7. **Conflict resolution:**
   - Conflict resolution skills are important for managing disagreements and problems in interpersonal relationships. This includes the ability to find constructive solutions and compromise.
8. **Resilience:**
   - Resilience refers to the ability to deal with challenges and setbacks without losing self-esteem. High resilience helps maintain positive social relationships.
9. **Self-presentation:**
   - The ability to present oneself appropriately involves the behavior, expression, and appearance to make a positive impression in various social situations.
10. **Self-confidence:**
    - Self-confidence is the ability to realistically know oneself and one's strengths and weaknesses. This promotes healthy self-esteem and self-confidence in social situations.

Social skills are crucial for personal and professional success, as well as well-being in social communities. It can be strengthened through learning, experience and conscious development. Individuals who have high social skills tend to have more satisfying relationships and are better able to cope with the demands of social life.

Speech therapy

Speech therapy is a medical-therapeutic specialty that deals with the diagnosis, prevention, counseling, therapy and rehabilitation of disorders of speech, speech, voice, swallowing and communication. Speech therapists, also known as speech therapists, are specialized professionals who support people of all ages whose communication skills are impaired. Some of the key features of speech therapy:

1. **Speech therapy:**
    - Speech therapy includes the treatment of speech disorders, such as delays in language development, grammar or vocabulary disorders.
2. **Speech therapy:**
    - People with pronunciation disorders, articulation problems, or stuttering may benefit from speech therapy. This includes training the speech muscles and improving pronunciation.
3. **Voice Therapy:**
    - Speech therapists treat voice disorders, which can include problems with voice quality, hoarseness, or other voice-related difficulties.
4. **Therapy for swallowing disorders (dysphagia):**
    - Individuals with swallowing disorders, whether due to neurological conditions, injuries, or other causes, may benefit from speech therapy to improve swallowing function.
5. **Prevention and counselling:**
    - Speech therapists offer preventive measures, counseling, and training to reduce risk factors for speech and communication disorders.
6. **Communication aids and training:**
    - Speech therapists can recommend techniques and tools to help communicate, especially in people with severe speech or language disorders.
7. **Working with different age groups:**
    - Speech therapists work with children, adolescents and adults who have different forms of

communication problems. This can range from promoting language development in children to rehabilitation after strokes or other neurological events in adults.
8. **Interdisciplinary cooperation:**
    - Speech therapists often work with other health professionals, such as doctors, psychologists, teachers, and occupational therapists, to ensure comprehensive care for their patients.

The work of a speech therapist usually begins with a comprehensive evaluation of the patient's individual skills and needs. Due to the variety of disorders treated by speech therapists and the different age groups they work with, their intervention is highly personalized and adapted to the specific needs of the individual.

Speech therapy can make a significant contribution to the quality of life of people who are faced with communication and speech disorders.

Spina bifida

Spina bifida is a congenital malformation in which the spine and spinal cord do not fully develop. The term "spina bifida" comes from Latin and means "split vertebra". It is a neural tube defect that occurs during embryonic development when the neural tube, from which the central nervous system is formed, does not close properly.

There are different forms of spina bifida, the most common of which are the following:

1. **Spina bifida occulta:** This is the mildest form and can often be asymptomatic. In this form, part of the spine does not close completely, but there is no bump or opening. Many people with spina bifida occulta do not experience any problems and may not even know they have the abnormality.
2. **Spina bifida cystica (open form):**
   - **Meningocele:** In this case, a bulge occurs through the open area in the spine, and the space between the spinal cord membranes (meninges) forms a fluid-filled cyst (meningocele). The spinal cord itself usually remains intact.
   - **Myelomeningocele:** This is the most serious form. Not only does a cyst occur, but the spinal cord and nerve tissue also leak out through the open spot in the spine. This can lead to various neurological problems, including paralysis and sensory impairment below the affected area.

The causes of spina bifida are not fully understood, but both genetic and environmental factors may play a role. Women who are pregnant or trying to become pregnant often receive folic acid recommendations, as a deficiency of folic acid is considered a risk factor for neural tube defects.

Treatment for spina bifida can vary depending on severity and symptoms and may include surgery, physical therapy, medications, and other therapeutic interventions. Early interventions and multidisciplinary care are often critical to improving quality of life and minimizing complications.

Strabismus

Strabismus, also known as strabismus, is an eye condition in which the eyes are not aligned parallel and therefore do not look at the same object at the same time. This occurs when the eye muscles are not properly coordinated, resulting in a disturbance in the position of the eyes.

There are several types of strabismus, including:

1. **Esotropia:** The eyes tend to squint inwards.
2. **Exotropia:** The eyes tend to squint outwards.
3. **Hypertropia:** One eye looks up, while the other is directed straight ahead.
4. **Hypotropia:** One eye looks down while the other is facing straight ahead.

Strabismus can be congenital or develop over time. In children, strabismus can cause vision problems because the brain has difficulty fusing the images from both eyes. This can lead to amblyopia, also known as "lazy eye," when an eye is not developed properly.

Treatment for strabismus can vary depending on the cause and severity. It can include eyeglasses, eye muscle training, prismatic corrections, or in some cases, surgical procedures. With early diagnosis and appropriate treatment, many people with strabismus can achieve normal visual function.

It is necessary to detect and treat strabismus early, especially in children, to ensure the best possible development of visual function.

Stress management

Stress management refers to the efforts and strategies people use to deal with life's challenges and minimize the impact of stress on their physical and mental health. Stress is a natural reaction of the body to stressful situations, but if it becomes chronic or not managed appropriately, it can lead to negative effects. Here are some strategies for coping with stress:

1. **Mindfulness and Meditation:**
    - Mindfulness practices, such as meditation and breathing exercises, can help calm the mind and keep the focus on the present moment. This can reduce stress and strengthen emotional resilience.
2. **Relaxation:**
    - Progressive muscle relaxation, autogenic training or yoga are examples of relaxation techniques that can help reduce physical tension and promote well-being.
3. **Regular physical activity:**
    - Exercising has been shown to have positive effects on mood and can reduce stress. It doesn't have to be intense training; even regular walking can be helpful.
4. **Healthy nutrition:**
    - A balanced diet helps to provide the body with the necessary nutrients and supports mental health. Stable blood sugar levels can help reduce stress.
5. **Adequate sleep:**
    - Sleep plays a crucial role in managing stress. Adequate and quality sleep promotes the recovery of the body and mind.
6. **Social support:**
    - Sharing with friends, family, or support groups can play an important role in managing stress. Sharing feelings and experiences can be relieving.

7. **Time management:**
   - Effective time management helps to organize everyday life and set priorities. This can help reduce the feeling of being overwhelmed.
8. **Relaxation through hobbies:**
   - Time for hobbies and activities that bring joy creates a balance to stress. It's important to regularly schedule time for things that are important to you personally.
9. **Self-reflection:**
   - The ability for self-reflection makes it possible to recognize one's own thought patterns and stress triggers. This forms the basis for targeted stress management.
10. **Professional Help:**
    - In some cases, it is advisable to seek professional help, especially if the stress persists or has a serious impact on the quality of life. Psychologists, therapists, or counselors can provide support.

Stress management is individual, and different people find different strategies effective. It is advisable to identify techniques that suit each person and regularly incorporate them into everyday life.

Supervision

Supervision is a professional process in which people are accompanied, supported and advised by qualified supervisors in their professional activities. This approach is applied in various professional contexts, including healthcare, social work, pedagogy, psychotherapy, and many others.

The main objectives of supervision are:

1. **Quality assurance:**
    - Through the continuous reflection and analysis of professional activities, the quality of work is to be ensured and improved.
2. **Personal Development:**
    - Supervision provides space for the personal and professional development of the supervisors. It allows for the exploration of personal values, beliefs, and professional goals.
3. **Problem solving:**
    - In supervision, professional challenges, ethical dilemmas or difficult situations can be discussed and solutions can be worked out together.
4. **Self-reflection:**
    - The supervisors are encouraged to reflect on their own patterns of thought and behavior. This fosters a deeper understanding of their work and fosters a professional attitude.
5. **Support:**
    - Supervision serves as a supportive space in which the supervisors can share their successes, but also difficulties and burdens. The supervisor provides support and feedback.
6. **Teamwork:**
    - In some contexts, group supervision is used to promote team collaboration and understand group dynamic processes.

There are different models and approaches in supervision, including:

- **Casuistic supervision:** The supervisors bring in specific cases or situations from their professional practice, which are then analysed together.
- **Case- or client-centered supervision:** The focus is on the needs and challenges of the client or patient.
- **Systemic supervision:** Here, the focus is on the interactions across the professional system, including the relationship between supervisor and supervisor.
- **Intervision groups:** Collegial supervision in which members of a group support and advise each other.

Supervision is especially important in professions where working with people is paramount, as it helps to improve the quality of services, promote professional development and prevent burnout. It is an established part of ongoing professional development in many industries.

Support Groups

Support groups are informal, community-based groups of people who meet regularly to support each other in overcoming common challenges, problems, or life situations. These groups provide a safe space where people with similar experiences or concerns can share their feelings, share resources, and encourage each other. Here is some information about support groups:

1. **Fellowship and Understanding:**
    - Support groups create a community of people who share similar experiences. This fosters understanding, empathy and solidarity among group members.
2. **Mutual assistance:**
    - The main goal of support groups is to offer mutual support. Members share their personal experiences, best practices, and advice to help each other overcome challenges.
3. **Emotional Support:**
    - Through the exchange of emotions and experiences, the group provides emotional support. This is especially important for people who are facing difficult life situations, illnesses or other stresses.
4. **Information and Resources:**
    - Support groups serve as a source of information. Members share information about best practices, local resources, professionals, and current developments related to their common concerns.
5. **Empowerment:**
    - The groups promote empowerment by encouraging members to actively participate in their own coping and make decisions that improve their quality of life.
6. **Anonymity and confidentiality:**
    - Support groups often provide a safe space for members to talk openly about their experiences, as anonymity and confidentiality are respected.

7. **Sense:**
    - The sense of community created by support groups can reduce feelings of isolation. Members often realize that they are not alone and that others are going through similar challenges.
8. **Self-reflection:**
    - By sharing stories and reflecting on the experiences of others, members can broaden their own perspectives and gain new insights.
9. **Practical tips and strategies:**
    - Support groups offer practical tips and proven strategies that members can use in their daily lives. This can range from proven coping mechanisms to concrete recommendations for action.
10. **Long-term support:**
    - Support groups can provide long-term support, even if members' living conditions or health conditions change over time. This promotes sustainable and continuous support.

Support groups can become an important complement to professional therapies and medical treatment. They are prevalent in various fields, including health, mental health, chronic illness, addiction, grief management, parenting, and much more. The diversity of support groups allows people to find support in relation to a wide range of challenges.

Support Reaction

The support response is a term used in child development and refers to the ability of a baby or toddler to hold their body upright or stabilize themselves when placed or placed on a surface. This response plays an important role in the development of upright posture and motor control.

There are different types of support reactions that occur in the course of development. Some of the most common are:

1. **Asymmetrical tonic neck reflexes (ATNR):** When the baby's head is turned in one direction, the arm on the same side stretches and the arm on the opposite side bends. This reaction usually occurs in infants around 2-4 months of age and then gradually disappears.
2. **Simultaneous Neck Reflex (STNR):** When the baby's head is tilted forward, the arms and legs straighten while the head is tilted back. This reaction usually occurs at 4-6 months of age.
3. **Labyrinth reaction:** This reaction occurs when the organ of balance in the inner ear is stimulated. For example, when the child is tilted forward, he stretches out his arms to keep his balance.
4. **Landau reflex:** When the baby lies on his stomach and the head is raised, the legs and back stretch upwards. This reaction usually occurs at 3-4 months of age.

Supportive responses are important milestones in the normal motor development of infants and young children. They help develop the muscle strength, coordination, and balance needed for later sitting, standing, and walking.

Supported communication

Assisted Communication (UK) is an educational and therapeutic concept that aims to help people with communication impairments express themselves better and actively participate in social life. This form of communication support is often used for people with developmental disabilities, autism, neurological disorders, cognitive impairment or motor impairments.

Here are some key features of assisted communication:

1. **Different means of communication:** Assisted communication uses a variety of communication aids and techniques to meet the needs of the individual. This includes pictorial symbols, signs, writing and drawing instruments, speech output devices, and other alternative or supportive means of communication.
2. **Individualization:** The approach of assisted communication is individually tailored to the abilities, preferences and needs of the person. It is important to identify the best methods and tools for the situation at hand.
3. **Training and support:** People who use assisted communication often need training to use the various means of communication effectively. Family members, caregivers, teachers, and therapists play a critical role in providing support and training.
4. **Promoting autonomy:** The goal of assisted communication is to promote the autonomy and self-determination of the person. This includes providing tools and strategies to facilitate communication in different areas of life.
5. **Combination of modalities:** A combination of different communication modalities is often used to increase versatility and effectiveness. For example, someone can use both pictorial symbols and gestures.

Assisted communication is designed not only to facilitate immediate communication, but also to improve social interaction, education, and participation in community life. The approach is dynamic and adapts to the changing needs and advances of the individual.

Tactile

"Tactile" refers to the sense of touch or tactile perception, the body's ability to receive information about its environment and objects through touch and pressure. The tactile sense plays an important role in human perception and interaction with the environment. Characteristics of tactile perception:

1. **Touch Sensitivity:**
   - Tactility includes sensitivity to touch and pressure. Some people are more sensitive, while others are less sensitive to touch.
2. **Tactile learning process:**
   - The tactile sense plays a key role in the learning process, especially in children. By touching and exploring objects, children learn a lot about their properties, textures and temperatures.
3. **Tactile Communication:**
   - Touch can be a form of non-verbal communication. A handshake, hug, or other tactile cues can express affection, support, or empathy.
4. **Tactile stimulation:**
   - Tactile stimulation can be calming or stimulating. Massages, touching different materials or tactile games can help to relax or activate.
5. **Tactile perception in people with disabilities:**
   - People with sensory processing disorders or neurological impairments may have different tactile perception patterns. Some may be hypersensitive and find touch overwhelming, while others may be hyposensitive and may be less sensitive to touch.
6. **Tactile stimuli in therapy:**
   - In various therapeutic approaches, such as occupational therapy, tactile stimuli can be used to promote sensory processing. This can be done by providing different textures, weights, or tactile exercises.

7. **Tactile orientation:**
    - Tactile stimuli also help with spatial orientation. People often use the tactile properties of surfaces to orient themselves in their environment.
8. **Tools for tactility:**
    - For people with visual impairments, tactile aids such as Braille or tactile maps are important tools for making information accessible.

In therapy, especially occupational therapy, tactile perception is often targeted to promote sensory integration and overall well-being, especially in people with developmental disabilities or neurological disorders.

Tactile perception

Tactile perception refers to the body's ability to sense and interpret touch. This aspect of sensory perception allows us to obtain information about the nature, temperature, pressure, vibrations and other tactile stimuli from our environment. Tactile perception plays a crucial role in everyday interaction with the world and is important for various aspects of daily life. It includes:

1. **Tactile sensitivity:** This refers to the ability to capture subtle tactile stimuli. Some people may have increased sensitivity to touch, while others may have decreased sensitivity.
2. **Tactile discrimination:** This is the ability to detect subtle differences in the texture, shape, and size of objects. It allows us to detect, for example, by touch whether an object is smooth or rough, warm or cold.
3. **Tactile localization:** This ability makes it possible to locate touch in specific parts of the body. For example, we can tell if we are being touched on the hand or arm.
4. **Tactile identification:** This refers to the ability to recognize objects or materials through touch without seeing them. An example would be recognizing an object in your hand without looking at it.
5. **Tactile consistency:** This concerns the ability to modulate pressure and force in the touch. It allows us to distinguish between gentle and firm touches.

Tactile perception plays an important role in children's development, especially in the area of fine motor skills and cognitive development. Tactile perception issues can affect various aspects of daily life, including self-care activities, school performance, and social interaction.

In occupational therapy, techniques and activities can be used to promote tactile perception and help people better adapt to their environment.

Tactile system

The tactile system, also known as somatosensory or tactile sense, is one of the body's sensory systems and refers to the perception of touch, pressure, vibration, temperature, and pain. It is an important part of the somatosensory system, which sends information about the state of the body and its environment to the brain.

Here are some features of the tactile system:

1. **Tactile receptors:** The skin contains a variety of tactile receptors that respond to different types of tactile stimuli. These include mechanoreceptors, thermoreceptors, and pain receptors.
2. **Tactile sensitivity:** Sensitivity to tactile stimuli varies in different parts of the body. For example, the fingertips are very sensitive, while the skin on the back is less sensitive.
3. **Tactile processing in the brain:** Information from the tactile system is transmitted via the peripheral nervous system to the spinal cord and then to the brain. The brain processes and interprets this information to enable a conscious perception of touch and other tactile stimuli.
4. **Tactile integration:** The tactile system often works with other sensory modalities to provide a comprehensive perception of one's environment and one's own body. For example, tactile perception can interact with visual perception to recognize objects.
5. **Tactile stimuli in everyday life:** Tactile stimuli are ubiquitous in daily life and play a role in activities such as touching, holding, grasping, writing, eating, and many other motor and social actions.

For some people, the tactile system can be hypersensitive or hyposensitive. Hypersensitivity can cause tactile stimuli to be overwhelming or unpleasant, while hyposensitivity can lead to a decreased perception of touch. These sensory processing differences can occur in various neurological or developmental disorders.

In occupational therapy, targeted tactile activities can be used to promote the perception and processing of tactile stimuli and to address any sensitivity issues.

Tetraparesis

Tetraparesis refers to paralysis or weakness that affects all four extremities (arms and legs). The term "tetraparesis" is composed of "tetra-" (Greek for "four") and "paresis" (partial paralysis or weakness).

This type of motor impairment can have various causes, including neurological disorders, traumatic spinal cord injuries, genetic disorders, or other medical conditions. Tetraparesis can range from mild to severe impairment, depending on the underlying cause and the extent of damage to the nervous system.

Some examples of conditions that can cause tetraparesis include:

1. **Spinal cord injury:** Trauma, often from spinal cord injury, can lead to spinal cord injury that causes tetraparesis.
2. **Neurodegenerative diseases:** Certain neurodegenerative diseases, such as amyotrophic lateral sclerosis (ALS) or spinal muscular atrophies, can cause progressive tetraparesis.
3. **Genetic disorders:** Some genetic disorders, such as Duchenne muscular dystrophy, can lead to progressive muscle weakness and tetraparesis.
4. **Stroke:** A serious stroke that affects the central nervous system can lead to tetraparesis.

The treatment and management of tetraparesis depends on the underlying cause. Physical therapy, occupational therapy, drug treatments, and supportive measures can be part of the treatment plan to improve mobility, maintain quality of life, and minimize complications. The prognosis may vary depending on the cause, severity, and therapeutic approach. Comprehensive medical examination and care for people with tetraparesis should be ensured to provide support.

Tone

The term "tone" refers to the state of tension of the muscles in the body. It is an important term in medicine, especially in the fields of neurology, orthopedics, rehabilitation and physiotherapy. Muscle tone describes how tight or relaxed the muscles are at any given moment.

There are two main types of muscle tone:

1. **Hypertension (increased muscle tone):** This condition occurs when the muscles are excessively tense and do not relax sufficiently. Hypertension can lead to stiffness, decreased range of motion, and pain. It can be caused by various factors, including neurological conditions such as spasticity in cerebral palsy or certain forms of muscle disease.
2. **Hypotonus (decreased muscle tone):** Hypotonus occurs when the muscles have less tension than usual. This can lead to weakness, instability, and decreased control over movements. Hypotension is often associated with neurological conditions such as certain forms of muscular dystrophy or brain damage.

Muscle tone is usually not constant, but can vary depending on activity, emotional state, and state of health. Normal tension allows the muscles to respond to stimuli, allow movement, and maintain an upright posture. Assessment of muscle tone is important for the diagnosis and management of various neurological and musculoskeletal conditions. Physical therapists and other health care providers can use targeted exercises and therapeutic approaches to influence muscle tone, especially in people with neurological disorders where hypertension or hypotension play a role.

Tone regulation

Tone regulation refers to the body's ability to regulate muscle tone, that is, to maintain and adjust tension in the muscles. Muscle tone is the degree of muscle tension or tightening when a muscle is at rest. Tone regulation is a complex process that is controlled by the interaction of nerves, muscles, and other tissues.

Tone regulation includes:

1. **Neurological control:** The nervous system plays a crucial role in regulating muscle tone. The motor neurons in the spinal cord and brain send signals to the muscles to control their contraction and relaxation.
2. **Feedback loops:** Muscle tone is regulated by feedback mechanisms that send information about the length and tension of the muscles to the nervous system. This sensory feedback allows for continuous adjustment of tone in different movement situations.
3. **Counterplay of muscles:** Antagonistic muscles often work together in pairs to make movement possible. When one muscle contracts (shortens), the opposite muscle relaxes, and vice versa. This interaction contributes to the regulation of muscle tone.
4. **Influence of hormones:** Hormones can also affect muscle tone. In particular, hormones such as adrenaline can cause a temporary increase in muscle tension.
5. **Tissue structures:** The elasticity of tendons, ligaments, and connective tissue around the muscles can affect muscle tone. Good elasticity and elasticity of these structures contribute to normal muscle tone.
6. **Coordination and posture:** Coordination of muscle activities and maintaining appropriate posture are crucial for tone regulation. Muscles need to work together to perform movements efficiently and maintain posture.

Abnormal changes in muscle tone can lead to various conditions, including hypertension (increased muscle tone) or hypotension (decreased muscle tone). These conditions can be due to neurological disorders, muscle disorders, or other health problems.

In rehabilitation, especially in physiotherapy and occupational therapy, tone regulation is often targeted to improve the movement skills and functioning of individuals affected by abnormal muscle tone changes. Therapeutic approaches may include exercise, stretching, sensory stimulation, and other interventions.

Transfer Skills

Transfer skills refer to the skills and abilities that allow a person to transfer from one activity or environment to another. These skills are crucial for self-reliance in daily life and play an important role in various fields such as healthcare, rehabilitation, and education. Transfer skills are often closely related to motor, cognitive, and emotional skills.

Here are some examples of transfer skills:

1. **Transfers in the physical sense:** Implementing skills to move from one place to another, whether it's moving from a chair to a wheelchair, transferring from a gurney to a healthcare exam table, or overcoming obstacles.
2. **Cognitive transfer skills:** The ability to transfer knowledge, skills, or strategies from one situation to another. This can mean, for example, applying learned concepts in different contexts.
3. **Emotional transfer skills:** The ability to transfer emotional regulation techniques or coping strategies from one situation to another. This is especially important to deal with various stressors and challenges.
4. **Transfer of skills in education:** The transfer of learning skills or techniques from one subject to another. For example, the ability to apply reading skills from English lessons to history lessons.
5. **Professional transfer skills:** In a professional context, this refers to the application of skills, knowledge, and experience from one job to another. This can include adapting to different work environments or tasks.
6. **Self-Care Transfer Skills:** The ability to apply personal hygiene, nutrition, or clothing care skills in different settings or stages of life.

Promoting transfer skills is often a goal in rehabilitation, especially in people with physical impairments or after an injury. Through targeted therapy and exercises, the ability to move effectively and safely in different contexts and to cope with tasks can be improved. In education, the promotion of transfer skills emphasizes the importance of learning skills that can be applied beyond the specific context in other areas of life.

Transfer Training

Transfer training is an important part of rehabilitation and refers to the targeted training of skills and techniques that allow a person to move safely from one place to another or move from one activity to the next. The focus is on promoting independence and safety in everyday movements. Here are some characteristics of transfer training:

1. **Movement Skills:**
    - Transfer skills include various movement skills, such as getting out of a chair, sitting down, moving from a bed to a wheelchair, or vice versa. The training focuses on performing these movements safely and efficiently.
2. **Tools and techniques:**
    - Training may include the use of assistive devices such as walkers, wheelchairs, or transfer boards. Specific techniques are also taught to make transfers safer, such as proper lifting and turning.
3. **Strength and endurance training:**
    - Effective transfer training often involves strength and endurance exercises to strengthen the muscles and develop the necessary endurance for safe transfers.
4. **Balance and stability:**
    - Balance and stability play an important role in transfers. Training may include exercises that improve balance and promote stability during movement.
5. **Advice on assistive devices:**
    - Depending on the individual needs of the person, transfer training can also include advice on the use of specific aids. This could include the use of gripping aids, seat cushions, or other assistive devices.
6. **Realistic situations:**
    - Transfer training should be conducted in real-life situations to ensure that the skills acquired can be directly transferred to the demands of daily life.

7. **Psychosocial support:**
    - The transfer process can be emotionally draining for some people, especially when they are recovering from injuries or surgery. Therefore, psychosocial support can be an integral part of training.
8. **Advanced Training:**
    - Advanced transfer training may also include tackling uneven terrain, getting in and out of vehicles, or tackling stairs, depending on individual goals and needs.

Transfer training is especially important for people who have difficulty moving due to injury, illness or impairment. Through targeted training, they can regain their independence and act more confidently in their environment. The exact approach depends on the specific needs and abilities of each person.

Trauma Therapy

Trauma therapy is a specialized area of psychotherapy that aims to help people who have lived through traumatic experiences process their emotions, thoughts, and behaviors. Traumatic events can take various forms, including physical or sexual violence, natural disasters, accidents, or other life-threatening situations. Trauma therapy is designed to mitigate the effects of these experiences and help those affected regain a stable emotional balance.

Some important approaches and methods in trauma therapy are:

1. **Stabilization:** In the first phases of trauma therapy, the focus is often on stabilization. This includes developing coping strategies to minimize current stresses, as well as promoting safety and control.
2. **Mindfulness and relaxation techniques:** Mindfulness and relaxation techniques can help reduce stress and calm the nervous system. This can lay the foundation for further therapeutic work.
3. **Confrontation with trauma memories:** Under the guidance of the therapist, the person can be gradually encouraged to deal with the traumatic memories. This can be done through techniques such as EMDR (Eye Movement Desensitization and Reprocessing) or Cognitive Processing of Trauma (CBT).
4. **Resource-oriented approaches:** Trauma therapy often incorporates resource-oriented approaches to promote the person's strengths and coping skills. This includes social support systems and self-care.
5. **Narrative approaches:** By telling their own story, the person can help integrate the trauma and find meaning. Narrative approaches can help to regain control over one's own life story.
6. **Body-oriented techniques:** Some therapists incorporate body-oriented techniques such as body awareness, breathwork, or somatic therapy to emphasize the connection between body and mind.

Trauma therapy is an individual process and not all methods are suitable for everyone. The therapeutic relationship plays a crucial role, and an experienced therapist can combine a variety of approaches to meet the person's needs. People interested in trauma therapy should consult with qualified professionals who have experience working with traumatized individuals.

Treatment plan

A treatment plan is a structured and documented plan that describes the specific steps and interventions to be carried out in a therapeutic process or health management procedure. Treatment plans are created in various areas of healthcare, including occupational therapy, to address the needs and goals of the patient or client. Considerations of a treatment plan:

1. **Diagnosis and evaluation:** The fundamental basis of a treatment plan is the diagnosis and evaluation of the individual's health status or therapeutic needs. This often includes a comprehensive examination, assessment of skills, limitations, and individual goals.
2. **Goals and objectives:** The treatment plan should set clear, measurable, and achievable goals for the patient or client. These goals should be based on the specific needs and diagnosis.
3. **Intervention strategies:** The plan should describe in detail what interventions or therapeutic measures will be used to achieve the defined objectives. This may include exercises, therapeutic activities, medications, counseling, or other methods.
4. **Frequency and duration:** The treatment plan should specify how often and for what period of time the interventions should be performed. This helps to monitor progress and ensure that treatment is appropriate and effective.
5. **Evaluation and adjustment:** Periodic assessments of progress should be established in the treatment plan to ensure that the interventions chosen are effective. If necessary, adjustments can be made to respond to changing needs or new developments.
6. **Communication and collaboration:** The treatment plan can also encourage the sharing of information between different healthcare providers and parties involved to ensure coherent and effective care.

The exact structure and content of a treatment plan can vary depending on the specific specialty and individual needs of the patient. In occupational therapy, the treatment plan is often created in close collaboration with the patient and other members of the healthcare team to provide comprehensive and patient-centered care.

Tremor

A tremor is a rhythmic, involuntary tremor or shaking of a part of the body. Tremor can have various causes and often occurs in the hands, but it can also affect other areas of the body, including the arms, legs, head, or torso. There are different types of tremor, which can vary depending on the cause and characteristics.

Here are some of the most common types of tremor:

1. **Essential tremor:** This is the most common form of tremor and often affects the hands. Essential tremor usually occurs during movement and may be genetic.
2. **Resting tremor:** This tremor occurs when the affected person is relaxed and not actively making a movement. One example is resting tremor in Parkinson's disease.
3. **Intention tremor:** This tremor occurs when a person makes targeted movements, such as touching the nose with their finger. Intention tremor can occur in various neurological disorders.
4. **Orthostatic tremor:** This tremor occurs when a person is standing and can cause them to tremble or feel unsafe. Sitting or lying down usually brings relief.
5. **Physiological tremor:** A mild tremor that occurs in most people and is often exacerbated by factors such as stress, caffeine consumption, or fatigue. Usually, physiological tremor is not pathological.
6. **Dystonic tremor:** This tremor occurs in people with dystonia, a neurological disorder that causes uncontrollable muscle contractions.

The causes of tremor can be varied, from genetic factors to neurological disorders to medications or metabolic disorders. The diagnosis and management of tremor requires a comprehensive evaluation by a doctor, preferably a neurologist. Treatment depends on the underlying cause and may include medication, physical therapy, or in some cases, surgery.

Vestibular perception

Vestibular perception refers to the body's ability to grasp and interpret information about spatial orientation and the sense of balance. This perception is based on signals from the vestibular system, a part of the inner ear responsible for detecting head movements, posture, and balance.

The vestibular system consists of the semicircular canals and the otolith organ in the inner ear. The semicircular canals respond to rotational movements of the head, while the otolith organ acts on linear accelerations and gravity. Together, these structures enable the perception of changes in head position and movement.

Some points of vestibular cognition are:

1. **Balance:** The vestibular system plays a key role in maintaining balance. It helps to respond to changes in body position and allows you to stand stably on your feet or balance yourself while moving.
2. **Spatial orientation:** Vestibular perception helps to understand spatial orientation in space. It helps to detect the orientation of the body in relation to gravity.
3. **Eye movements:** Vestibular perception is closely related to the control of eye movements. This makes it possible to keep the gaze stable when the head is in motion and to focus on visual stimuli.

Problems with vestibular perception can lead to balance problems, dizziness and coordination problems. Occupational therapists and physical therapists often use specific exercises and techniques to promote vestibular perception and help people better handle sensory information about their spatial position and movement.

Especially in people with diseases of the vestibular system or after injuries that affect balance, rehabilitation can be aimed at improving vestibular perception and optimizing functioning in everyday life.

Visual perception

Visual perception refers to the ability of the visual system to absorb, interpret, and organize visual stimuli from the environment. It is a crucial aspect of perception and plays a central role in various areas of daily life. Visual perception encompasses various processes that work together to provide a meaningful interpretation of visual stimuli. Here are some features of visual perception:

1. **Form perception:** The ability to recognize and distinguish shapes is a fundamental aspect of visual perception. This includes the identification of objects regardless of their size, location or orientation.
2. **Color perception:** The visual perception of colors makes it possible to distinguish different wavelengths of light. This aspect plays an important role in the identification of objects and the interpretation of visual stimuli.
3. **Depth perception:** The visual perception of depth makes it possible to understand the spatial arrangement of objects. This includes skills such as detecting distances and distinguishing between near and distant objects.
4. **Motion perception:** The ability to track and interpret movement is another important aspect of visual perception. This plays a role in orienting oneself in space and perceiving changes in the environment.
5. **Visual integration:** The ability to process multiple visual stimuli at the same time and integrate them into a coherent perception is crucial. This allows for a comprehensive interpretation of the visual environment.

In occupational therapy, targeted exercises and interventions can be used to promote visual perception, especially when it is impaired due to developmental disorders, injuries or illnesses. This can help to improve independence in everyday activities and increase quality of life.

Water aerobics

Water aerobics is a therapeutic form of exercise that is performed in the water and can be an important part of occupational therapy. It is based on the physical properties of the water, in particular buoyancy, resistance and temperature.

This form of gymnastics offers a variety of benefits for people who suffer from various health challenges or impairments. These include, for example, patients with muscular or orthopaedic problems, neurological diseases or rheumatic complaints.

The buoyancy of the water reduces body weight, which makes it easier to perform movements and relieve joints. At the same time, water resistance provides a gentle way to strengthen muscles and improve mobility. The temperature of the water helps to relieve muscle tension and promote blood circulation.

In occupational therapy, water aerobics can be customized to take into account the patient's specific goals and needs. The exercises can be varied, from simple movements to more complex exercises that promote coordination and balance. Water aerobics is often used in conjunction with other occupational therapy approaches to provide comprehensive therapeutic support.

Word-finding disorder

A word-finding disorder refers to difficulty recalling or finding words from the vocabulary while speaking or writing. This can manifest itself in various forms, including:

- **Tip-of-the-tongue phenomenon:** The person knows what word they want to use but can't remember it right away. It feels like the word is "on the tip of the tongue."
- **Paraphasia:** The use of words that sound or look similar instead of the desired word.
- **Paraphrasing:** The person uses descriptions or descriptive words instead of the exact term.

Word-finding disorders can have various causes, including neurological diseases such as stroke, dementia, brain injuries or neurodegenerative diseases.

Youth welfare

Youth welfare is a system of measures and services that aims to promote, support and protect children and young people in their individual development. The focus is on the well-being and needs of young people. Youth welfare is an important part of social services and includes various facilities, programmes and professional support. Further basic information on youth welfare:

1. **Prevention and support:** Youth welfare focuses on preventive measures and the promotion of the positive development of children and young people. This includes programmes to strengthen social skills, leisure activities, educational projects and similar measures.
2. **Educational assistance:** In cases where young people and their families need special support, educational assistance can be offered. These include, for example, outpatient educational assistance, home education, foster families, socio-pedagogical family assistance and intensive socio-pedagogical individual care.
3. **Child and youth work:** Youth welfare also includes activities of child and youth work, which includes extracurricular education, leisure activities and cultural activities. Youth centres, holiday camps, sports clubs and similar facilities offer space for personal development and social integration.
4. **Protection against neglect and abuse:** An important task of youth welfare is to protect children and young people from neglect, abuse and other forms of endangerment. This includes measures for early detection, intervention and support of affected families.
5. **Advice and support:** Youth welfare institutions offer counselling services for children, young people and their families. This can include help in personal crises, support with school problems, or parenting issues.
6. **Youth social work:** Youth welfare also includes measures for the integration of disadvantaged young people into education and work. This includes career orientation,

qualification measures and accompanying socio-educational support.
7. **Participation of children and young people:** The participation of children and young people in decisions that affect them is a principle of youth welfare. Participation should promote their self-determination and personal responsibility.
8. **Family support services:** Youth welfare services also offer family support services that aim to strengthen and support families in their educational task. These include, for example, parenting courses, family counselling and support in coping with everyday problems.

Youth welfare is regulated by law in many countries and is subject to certain quality standards and ethical principles. In Germany, for example, the Child and Youth Welfare Act (SGB VIII) is the legal basis for youth welfare.

IMPRESSUM
Information according to § 5 TMG:
Markus Gohlke
c/o IP Management #16265
Ludwig-Erhard-Str. 18
20459 Hamburg
Contact:
E-mail: elcamondobeach@gmail.com
Phone: +491751555847
Imprint: Independently published

www.ingramcontent.com/pod-product-compliance
Lightning Source LLC
Chambersburg PA
CBHW050157230526
45470CB00001B/128